AF690944

FOOD SAFETY
THE IMPLICATIONS OF CHANGE FROM PRODUCERISM TO CONSUMERISM

Edited by

JAMES J. SHERIDAN, Ph.D.

Head, Food Safety Department
Teagasc, The National Food Centre
Dunsinea, Castleknock
Dublin 15, Ireland

MICHAEL O'KEEFFE, Ph.D.

Food Safety Department
Teagasc, The National Food Centre
Dunsinea, Castleknock
Dublin 15, Ireland

MARK ROGERS, Ph.D.

Department of Zoology
University College Dublin
Belfield, Dublin 4, Ireland

FOOD & NUTRITION PRESS, INC.
TRUMBULL, CONNECTICUT 06611 USA

Copyright © 1998 by

FOOD & NUTRITION PRESS, INC.
Trumbull, Connecticut 06611 USA

All rights reserved. No part of this publication may be reproduced, stored in a retrieval system or transmitted in any form or by any means: electronic, electrostatic, magnetic tape, mechanical, photocopying, recording or otherwise, without permission in writing from the publisher.

Library of Congress Catalog Card Number: 98-074928
ISBN: 0-917678-48-6

CONTRIBUTORS

THOMAS ARNOLD, Assistant Secretary, Department of Agriculture and Food, Agriculture House, Kildare Street, Dublin 2, Ireland.

HENK BEKMAN, IKB Programme Coordinator, Product Board for Livestock Meat and Eggs, Sir Winston Churchilllaan 275, Postbus 5805, 2280 HV Rijswijk, The Netherlands.

KEVIN BRENNAN, Industrial Liaison Officer, The National Food Centre, Teagasc, Dunsinea, Castleknock, Dublin 15, Ireland.

ROBERT L. BUCHANAN, Research Leader, U.S. Food and Drug Administration, 200 "C" Street, Washington, DC 20204 USA.

JOHN D. COLLINS, Professor, Faculty of Veterinary Medicine, University College Dublin, Ballsbridge, Dublin 4, Ireland.

CATHAL A. COWAN, Senior Research Officer, Food Marketing Research Group, The National Food Centre, Teagasc, Dunsinea, Castleknock, Dublin 15, Ireland.

PATRICK DALY, Senior Research Officer, Quality Services Department, The National Food Centre, Teagasc, Dunsinea, Castleknock, Dublin 15, Ireland.

LIAM DOWNEY, Director, Teagasc, 19 Sandymount Avenue, Ballsbridge, Dublin 4, Ireland.

THOMAS DOYLE, Head, Quality Services Department, The National Food Centre, Teagasc, Dunsinea, Castleknock, Dublin 15, Ireland.

CAROLINE GILL, Chief Executive, Consumers' Association of Ireland, 45 Upper Mount Street, Dublin 2, Ireland.

THOMAS R. GORMLEY, Head, Consumer Foods Department, The National Food Centre, Teagasc, Dunsinea, Castleknock, Dublin 15, Ireland.

CECILY KELLEHER, Professor, Department for Health Promotion, University College Galway, Galway, Ireland.

ORLA KENNEDY, Research Officer, Food Safety Department, The National Food Centre, Teagasc, Dunsinea, Castleknock, Dublin 15, Ireland.

DAVID MCCONNELL, Professor, Department of Genetics, University of Dublin, Trinity College, Dublin 2, Ireland.

ROBERT M. MCCRACKEN, Deputy Chief Veterinary Officer, Department of Agriculture for Northern Ireland, Dundonald House, Upper Newtownards Road, Belfast BT4 3SB, Northern Ireland.

JAMES D. MCNEIL, Head, Centre for Veterinary Drug Residues, Canadian Food Inspection Agency, Saskatoon, Saskatchewan, Canada, 57N 2R3.

ARTHUR J. MILLER, Research Leader, U.S. Food and Drug Administration, 200 "C" Street, Washington, DC 20204 USA.

ALISTAIR MORTON, Group Director of Technical Affairs, Greencore Group plc., St Stephen's Green House, Earlsfort Terrace, Dublin 2, Ireland.

MICHAEL O'KEEFFE, Principal Research Officer, Department of Food Safety, The National Food Centre, Teagasc, Dunsinea, Castleknock, Dublin 15, Ireland.

THOMAS P. OSCAR, Research Food Technologist, Agricultural Research Service, Microbial Food Safety Research Unit, United States Department of Agriculture, 1124 Princess Anne, Maryland 21853, USA.

WILLIAM PATERSON, Technical Manager, Tesco Ireland, Gresham House, Marine Road, Dun Laoghaire, Co. Dublin, Ireland.

T. HUGH PENNINGTON, Professor of Bacteriology, University of Aberdeen, Medical School Buildings, Foresthill, Aberdeen, Scotland AB 25 2 ZD.

PETER PRENDERGAST, Director, Consumer Policy and Consumer Health Protection, European Commission Directorate General XXIV, Food and Veterinary Office, Trident House, Rock Hill, Blackrock, Co. Dublin, Ireland.

MARK ROGERS, Lecturer, Department of Zoology, University College Dublin, Belfield, Dublin 4, Ireland.

JAMES J. SHERIDAN, Head, Food Safety Department, The National Food Centre, Teagasc, Dunsinea, Castleknock, Dublin 15, Ireland.

JAMES L. SMITH, Research Leader, Microbial Food Safety Research Unit, Eastern Regional Research Centre, Agricultural Research Service, United States Department of Agriculture, 600 East Mermaid Lane, Wyndmoor, Philadelphia, Pennsylvania, USA.

DAVID M. TAYLOR, Principal Research Scientist, Neuropathogenesis Unit, Institute for Animal Health, West Mains Road, Edinburgh EH9 3JF, Scotland.

PREFACE

In recent years there has been a dramatic change with respect to concerns regarding food safety. Of particular note is the legal change that consumers have a right to be sold safe food and that the primary producer is now part of the process which must guarantee the delivery of safe products. The rise in consumerism has been strengthened by the introduction of new legislation on the production of safe food, and in particular by the setting up of a new Directorate General — DG XXII to deal with all matters affecting consumer safety in the European Union. This recognition of the rights of consumers in relation to food safety comes against a background of increasing concerns regarding bovine spongiform encephalopathy (BSE), *E. coli* O157:H7 and genetically modified organisms (GMOs).

Consumers want to know what controls are in place to reduce the risk from pathogens and if these controls actually work. While Hazard Analysis of Critical Control Points (HACCP) has been available as a means of controlling the spread of contaminants, both microbial and chemical, it is important that it is used by industry in a manner that offers the consumer a means of protection. In this regard the implementation of food safety assurance at farm level is seen as a priority, and efforts to implement such systems are on-going and are seen as vital in combating the spread of diseases of animal origin to foods.

This book contains papers presented at a conference held in Dublin on 6th and 7th November 1997. The objective of the conference was to highlight the changes in consumer attitudes to food safety. This is against the background that food production issues and concerns were increasingly seen as having undue influence on the implementation of food controls and regulations.

The conference addressed some of the issues involved in consumer concerns on food safety and the processes that are in place or need to be put in place to deal with any problems arising.

The conference was organised by Dr. J.J. Sheridan and Dr. M. O'Keeffe of The National Food Centre, Dr. Mark Rogers of University College Dublin, and supported financially by the European Union and by Teagasc.

JAMES J. SHERIDAN
MICHAEL O'KEEFFE
MARK ROGERS

CONTENTS

CHAPTER PAGE

Session I. Retailer and Regulatory Perspectives
Chairman: Dr. L. Downey

Session II. Food Safety Issues
Chairman: Professor C. Kelleher

Session III. Food Safety Control
Chairman: Professor D. Collins

Session IV. Systems for Food Safety Assurance
Chairman: Dr. A. Morton

CHAPTER 1

FOOD SAFETY ISSUES OF CONSUMER CONCERN

CAROLINE GILL

Consumers' Association of Ireland
45, Upper Mount Street, Dublin 2

ABSTRACT

For many years, the Consumers' Association of Ireland has highlighted problems connected with food safety, and has pressed for the removal of the responsibility for the supervision of food production from the Department of Agriculture and Food. Because the primary focus of the Department of Agriculture and Food was in advocating and asserting the interests of the producers, i.e., farmers and agri-business, the interests of consumers were frequently seen as, at best, a secondary consideration. Following the public concern created by the Creutzfeldt-Jakob Disease (CJD)/Bovine Spongiform Encephalopathy (BSE) issue, the Government announced the removal of food safety supervision from the Department of Agriculture and Food and the creation of a legislatively independent Food Safety Authority under the Minister of Health. Despite the serious consequences of delay in the establishment of this new organisation, progress on enacting the necessary legislation and bringing the new agency into being has been surprisingly slow. As these structural changes are being made, cases of BSE continue to occur in Ireland, further reducing local and international confidence in Irish beef. At home, consumers continue to question the safety of Irish beef, while abroad, loss of sales to Russia and Egypt present just two examples of the loss of international confidence in one of Ireland's major export products.

The Consumer Association of Ireland is calling on the Government to speed up all aspects of the establishment of the Food Safety Authority.

INTRODUCTION

This paper examines a number of consumer concerns in relation to food safety, particularly the concept that food production should be consumer-focused. Until very recently the Department of Agriculture and Food and its successive ministers, saw their primary role as advocating and asserting the interests of producers, farmers and agri-business, while the interests of the consumer were seen to be of secondary importance. The needs of consumers should, however, be of central importance, as it is in everybody's interest, including producers, to have an excellent reputation in meeting consumer requirements.

Ireland needs to create an international centre of excellence in consumer food protection. It is important for the consumer, and the producer and the good name of Irish food, that these needs are met in order to maintain or enhance the wider reputation of Irish food.

FOOD SAFETY AUTHORITY OF IRELAND

Following public concern created by BSE, antibiotic residues in pork, nitrate residues in vegetables, and *Salmonella* in chicken, the Government announced the removal of responsibility for food safety inspection from the Department of Agriculture and Food and the formation of an independent Food Safety Authority under the Minister for Health. At present, however, progress in the development of the Food Safety Authority of Ireland (FSAI) is very slow. The new agency needs to be established as soon as possible, with the necessary statutory basis, adequate resources, and staffing. When these are in place, the FSAI will be able to undertake its role in the inspection of food and food premises, the development of systems for the surveillance of food related disease in humans, livestock and food and the establishment of related educational and advisory roles. A national scheme for the surveillance of foodborne disease must be established. At present it is not possible to effectively trace and investigate any outbreak of foodborne disease. Adequate surveillance should be able to identify contaminated products and ensure their removal from the market, as well as establishing the causative pathogens and products, and targeting appropriate intervention. To serve as an early warning system, this surveillance centre will require the effective combination of the skills of doctors, veterinarians, food scientists and information specialists.

CONSUMER CONCERNS

Information

Consumers are concerned that adequate information about food is not available, nor do they know if important facts about food are being withheld. For example, when it became clear that antibiotic residue levels in pork were very high, the Department of Agriculture and Food informed producers, but did not inform consumers. The Consumers' Association of Ireland (CAI), in their report, released this information to the Irish public. Although the public pay for analysis of samples from food service establishments, the results of such tests are not readily available to consumers. Frequently, the information which does emerge into the public arena may be a year out of date. More current information should be comprehensively and rapidly available, by means of the Internet or the production of a weekly one page briefing of the type used by the police to circulate data on road traffic injuries and fatalities. Such a leaflet on food safety would be of great benefit to consumers and should not be difficult to provide if the relevant authorities were willing.

Food Labelling

Consumers are also concerned about inadequate labelling of food products. As choice increases and consumers become more aware of healthy eating they want more comprehensive and accurate information about the food on offer. For example, unpasteurised cheese does not have to be labelled as such, and there is no requirement for the manufacturer to indicate that unpasteurised cheese can pose an increased risk to some consumer groups including the elderly or expectant mothers. Consumers have wider concerns in relation to products being described as "natural", "wholesome", "light", "low", "traditional", "pure", etc., and are pressing for greater control of such nutritional and other claims, at national and European Union (EU) level.

National Beef Quality Assurance Scheme

Although there are a number of activities which could form elements of a future national beef quality assurance scheme, an acceptably comprehensive system is not yet in operation. Some of the current local schemes may be motivated more by sales than quality, and their multiplicity causes confusion and increased scepticism. Consumers need an independent, multidisciplinary, certifiable, auditable scheme, which is free of vested interests and which has a priority of advising and informing consumers. Consumers believe that a "two-tier" inspection system is operating in Ireland and that the export market is being better served and protected than the home market. Some abattoirs are still not under proper control, and ten local authorities are not taking responsibility for abattoirs in their regions.

Animal Diseases

There are also concerns in relation to a number of animal-related diseases. There are indications that cases of brucellosis are increasing, and very little progress is being made in the eradication of bovine tuberculosis (TB) (Anon. 1997). Although consumers are aware that it is important to eradicate TB from the national herd, they are dissatisfied that meat inspectors are spending large amounts of their time on this single priority. Perhaps meat inspectors should be working on the wider range of problems related to organisms such as *E. coli, Campylobacter* and *Salmonella,* to ensure that the farmyard is kept out of the abattoir.

Food Handlers and the Food Chain

Food handlers do not have to undergo mandatory training in food hygiene. A CAI survey of food hygiene in fish processing found ignorance of the rules of basic hygiene, products not being hygienically processed, and storage temperatures that were frequently unsatisfactory. Education in, and application of, good food hygiene, is the responsibility of everybody at the four main stages of the food chain.

(1) Farmers must send clean, healthy stock, free of pathogens and chemical residues, to the abattoir. If they don't, infected animals will enter the system and the final product may be contaminated.
(2) Food plants should apply HACCP procedures using modern technology and scientific testing to maintain product quality and safety during processing.
(3) Staff managing and handling food at the retail stage should be subject to mandatory training, to prevent frequent problems in relation to unsatisfactory hygiene, poor temperature control, etc.
(4) Finally, consumers must recognise their very important role in food hygiene and the need for education in the proper storage, preparation and cooking of food.

RECOMMENDATIONS

When the interests of the consumer are properly protected, everybody wins. It is important to recognise this fact, and to ensure high levels of food safety, not just for the benefit of Irish consumers, but as a vital means of maintaining and enhancing the contribution of Irish food exports to overall economic activity.

The protection of the consumer interest is important not just for the Irish consumer but for the good name of Irish food, the export of which is such an important component of our economic activity.

CHAPTER 2

IRISH AND EUROPEAN CONSUMER VIEWS ON FOOD SAFETY

CATHAL COWAN

Teagasc, The National Food Centre
Dunsinea, Castleknock, Dublin 15, Ireland

ABSTRACT

Results from two consumer surveys are presented. In the first, an EU FAIR (European Union Food, Agriculture and Industrial Research Programme), supported project, three-thousand consumers (500 in each of six countries, Germany, Italy, Britain, Spain, Sweden and Ireland) were surveyed, in March 1997, on their attitudes to the quality and safety of three meats, beef, pork and chicken. This paper deals with the safety aspects of the survey. Many consumers in all six countries said they were eating less beef and more chicken. Overall the Spanish and Irish appeared to be the most concerned about the safety of meat, the British were somewhat less concerned. While many were confident that the food in shops is safe there was a sizeable minority who believed the contrary. When looking for information on the safety of meat, butchers, whether independent or in supermarkets, are the group most trusted by consumers. In terms of consumer concerns, about 60 percent of beef consumers were very concerned about hormones, BSE (Bovine Spongiform Encephalopathy), antibiotics and bacteria. Pork consumers had similar levels of concern as beef consumers about bacteria, antibiotics and hormones. For chicken there was a higher level of concern about bacteria (Salmonella) *(68% were very concerned) and similar levels of concern to pork and beef for the other issues. Generally, fat was the issue of least concern for all three meats. Freshness was considered to be relatively the most helpful of 7 factors used for assessing safety of meat. The country of origin and what the animal was fed were also considered to be relatively helpful. Factors considered to be relatively less helpful were price and the name of the producer. In the second study, over 1200 pre-leaving certificate Irish school children participated in autumn 1996 in a national survey assessing young people's attitudes to meat. Half of the respondents agreed with the view that eating beef means increasing the risk of getting CJD (Creutzfeldt-Jakob Disease). Those who agreed were more likely to be less frequent eaters of beef and to have reduced their meat consumption in the post BSE period. It was found also that females were more likely to eat less meat than males and to have reduced beef consumption. The implications of some of the findings of these two surveys are discussed.*

INTRODUCTION

The impact of consumer concerns on meat consumption is of particular interest to the food industry. In Ireland, for example, the official statistics for the last 10 years show that beef consumption has steadily declined (Table 1). On the other hand poultry consumption has increased. Beef consumption declined by 13% in 1996 compared with the 1995 level. The long-term decline originated with concern about fat and continued with reports about growth promoters. In more recent years BSE has become an additional risk factor for consumers. Other factors, not necessarily associated with safety may also be involved. These include animal welfare, taste and convenience. Recent reports claiming an association of animal products with cancers is another difficulty. This research aims to measure consumer perceptions on a number of food safety issues and to look at their impact on consumption.

TABLE 1.
CONSUMPTION OF BEEF, PIGMEAT AND POULTRY IN IRELAND (kgs/person)

Year	Beef	Pigmeat*	Poultry	Total (all meats)
1986	22.3	34.5	18.4	81.9
1987	21.2	33.6	19.8	81.6
1988	19.3	35.4	20.7	82.1
1989	18.8	35.6	19.6	81.4
1990	17.9	35.2	21.6	82.9
1991	17.3	38.0	23.3	86.8
1992	17.1	37.2	23.5	85.9
1993	17.2	35.9	25.5	87.4
1994	15.7	36.6	27.8	88.2
1995	14.6	37.8	30.4	90.4
1996	12.7	37.8	31.0	89.2

**Pork and bacon.*
Source: Meat Supply Balances, various issues, Central Statistics Office, Cork, Ireland

METHODOLOGY

Objectives

There are 3 objectives of the EU FAIR study. The first is to identify consumers' perceptions on the quality and safety of beef, pork and chicken. The second is to describe how quality policy is operated in each country. The third is to relate consumers' expectations on food quality and safety to quality management programmes with the aim of developing more consumer-oriented quality policies. This paper deals with the first objective.

The study with Irish adolescents (16-17 years of age) deals with a number of topics on attitudes to meat. There is evidence from the study that factors other than safety are impacting on meat consumption. These include animal welfare, taste, vegetarianism, convenience and healthiness. The main aim of this part of the paper is to examine the relationship between attitudes to CJD and beef consumption changes.

Materials and Methods

The FAIR survey was carried out in March 1997. Three-thousand consumers (500 in each of six countries, Germany, Italy, Britain, Spain, Sweden and Ireland) were interviewed on their perceptions of the quality and safety of three meats, beef, pork and chicken. The sample was drawn at random from respondents where at least one member of their household eats one or more of the three meats. The approach used is based on perceived quality as defined by Steenkamp (1989) i.e. "the way consumers form judgements about the quality of a product on the basis of incomplete information". In this case safety perceptions rather than quality perceptions were measured by way of 5 point scales. While there have been a number of studies in individual countries this study has the benefit of being undertaken in 6 countries. It may be compared with a US study (Vosen *et al.* 1992) on consumer attitudes to food safety which found that about 61% of all consumers were very concerned about the safety of all foods they consume. Some 42% believed beef was very safe versus 18% who expressed a higher level of concern about red meat safety than any other food. The comparable figures for higher level of concern for fish & seafood and poultry safety were 33% and 17%, respectively, indicating beef was more acceptable than these products in safety terms. Americans, in 1992, were also more concerned about bacteria and fat in beef than hormones and antibiotics.

Results are presented for consumer attitudes regarding concerns about meat, the helpfulness of a number of factors for assessing the safety of meat, attitudes on food safety and who or what consumers most trust in looking for information on the safety of meat. Further analysis was used to establish whether the differences in ranking of concerns were statistically significant. The Wilcoxon signed rank test was undertaken for each pair of concerns. Concerns not statistically different are grouped together in the tables of results. Similarly helpfulness factors that are not statistically different are grouped together.

In the second study, as part of an EU Structural Funds project, over 1200 pre-leaving certificate Irish students participated in autumn 1996 in a national survey assessing young people's attitudes to meat. Results are presented for two safety-related statements, the respondents beliefs about CJD and their attitude to food in general. Finally, their opinion on how much confidence they have in what various organisations and companies have to say about meat-related issues was ascertained.

EU CONSUMER PERCEPTIONS ON MEAT SAFETY

Ranking of Concerns

Consumers were asked how concerned or unconcerned they were personally about the following issues when buying fresh beef, pork and chicken: growth promoters (hormones), antibiotics, fat or cholesterol, *Salmonella* or other bacteria, and BSE (beef only). Five point measurement scales ("very concerned" to "not at all concerned") were used. Table 2 shows the proportion of consumers for the six countries combined who were "very concerned". The proportion of consumers who were "very concerned" varied between 56 and 62% for most issues, except for *Salmonella* in chicken at 68% and for fat/cholesterol at 34-39%. Data on the range (lowest to highest) show that the level of concern varies considerably between countries for each issue.

TABLE 2.
CONSUMER CONCERNS - SIX COUNTRY AVERAGES

Concern	Proportion of consumers (%) "very concerned"					
	Beef		Pork		Chicken	
	average	range	average	range	average	range
hormones	60	(52-76)	57	(44-67)	56	(47-67)
antibiotics	57	(45-72)	57	(42-68)	55	(43-71)
BSE	62	(51-72)	-		-	
bacteria/*Salmonella*	58	(46-73)	60	(46-71)	68	(48-81)
fat/cholesterol	37	(20-47)	39	(24-57)	34	(21-46)

For presentation of the detailed results by country the average scores for each concern were calculated and the concerns were then ranked within each country.

Beef. The within-country groups, taking the statistical analysis into account, are shown in Table 3. Hormones were in the group of issues of most concern in all countries. Antibiotics were of equal concern in 5 countries, being of slightly lower concern to Spanish consumers. BSE, hormones, antibiotics and bacteria/*Salmonella* were perceived to be of equal concern in the U.K. and Sweden. BSE was regarded with the same high level of concern as hormones and antibiotics in Germany and Italy, while bacteria/*Salmonella* were of the same concern in Ireland. The latter issue was of somewhat lower concern to German, Spanish and Italian consumers. Fat or cholesterol was of least concern in all six countries.

TABLE 3.
GROUPING OF BEEF CONCERNS WITHIN EACH COUNTRY
(A = highest level of concern, D = lowest)

Concern	Ireland	United Kingdom	Sweden	Germany	Spain	Italy
hormones	A	A	A	A	A	A
antibiotics	A	A	A	A	B	A
fat or cholesterol	C	B	B	C	D	B
bacteria/*Salmonella*	A	A	A	B	B	B
BSE	B	A	A	A	C	A

Note: In this and similar subsequent tables concerns not statistically different are grouped together.

The detailed results by country for concern about hormones in beef and BSE are shown in Fig. 1 and 2. They illustrate considerable levels of concern in all countries. They also illustrate the varying levels of concern between the countries. In the case of hormones in beef, more consumers in Spain and Ireland were concerned than in the other countries; those "very concerned" varied from 47% in the UK to 73% and 76% in Spain and Ireland, respectively. In the case of BSE, although Irish consumers were less concerned about BSE than they were about antibiotics and hormones, they indicated greater concern about BSE than consumers in other countries. Levels of "very concerned" varied from 51% for British consumers to 72% for Irish consumers.

Pork. The within-country groups for pork, based on average scores and statistical analysis, are shown in Table 4. In Ireland, Sweden and Spain, *Salmonella* or other bacteria, antibiotics and hormones, had equally high concern scores. For the UK bacteria/*Salmonella* were of more concern than hormones and antibiotics while the reverse applied for Germany. Fat or cholesterol causes the least concern in five of the six countries. The exception was Italy where differences in the degree of concern were not significant for all the issues studied.

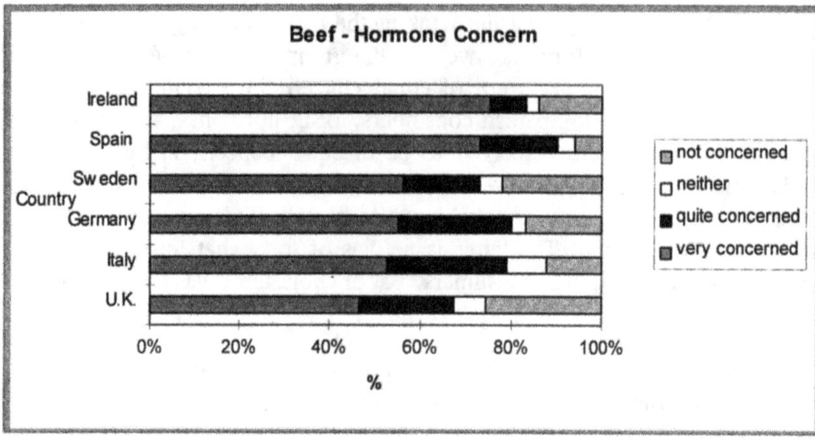

*Chi square[1] = 186***, n = 2449*

FIG. 1. CONCERN ABOUT HORMONES WHEN BUYING BEEF

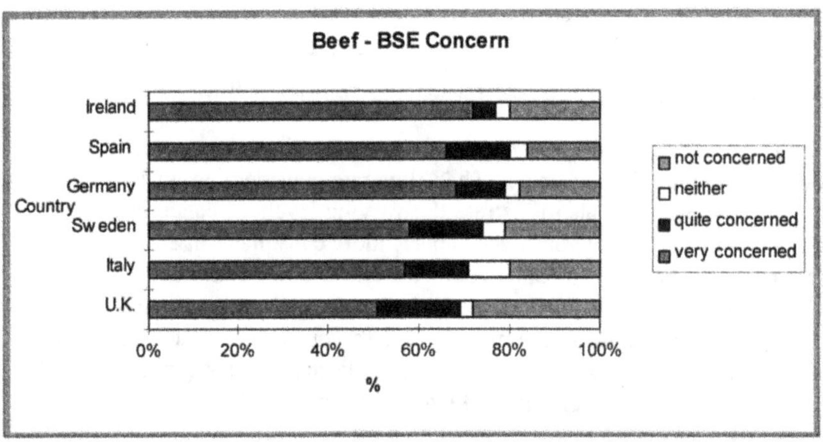

*Chi square = 104.9 ***, n = 2449*

FIG. 2. CONCERN ABOUT BSE WHEN BUYING BEEF

[1] Chi square tests were used to test for significance for this and all similar charts or tables. For presentation purposes the low proportion of "don't knows" are included with those who were "neither concerned nor unconcerned". Those "not very concerned" and "not at all concerned" are also combined in "not concerned". There were significant differences in scoring between consumers in the six countries for all results presented.

TABLE 4.
GROUPING OF PORK CONCERNS WITHIN EACH COUNTRY
(A = highest, C = lowest)

Concern	Ireland	United Kingdom	Sweden	Germany	Spain	Italy
hormones	A	B	A	A	A	A
antibiotics	A	B	A	A	A	A
fat or cholesterol	B	C	B	C	B	A
bacteria/*Salmonella*	A	A	A	B	A	A

Detailed results by country for concern about antibiotics in pork are shown in Fig. 3. They illustrate considerable levels of concern in all countries, but, also, the varying levels of concern between the countries. Italian and UK consumers were the least concerned with 42 and 52% being very concerned, respectively. Irish consumers were the most concerned with 68% being very concerned.

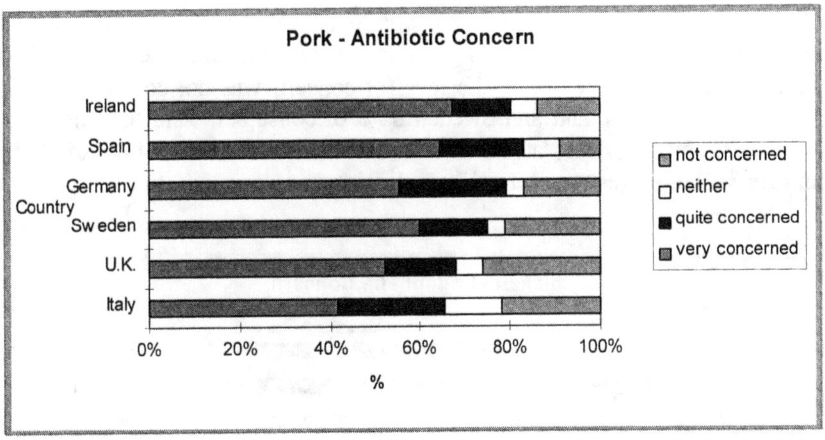

Chi square = 121.4 ***, n = 2374

FIG. 3. CONCERN ABOUT ANTIBIOTICS WHEN BUYING PORK

Chicken. The within-country groups for chicken are shown in Table 5. For chicken a similar pattern emerged in all countries. Bacteria/*Salmonella* was in the top group of concerns in all six countries. In Spain hormones, and in Italy both hormones and antibiotics, were of equal concern as bacteria/*Salmonella*. The main difference between countries was between hormones and antibiotics as their second greatest concern with antibiotics generally of more concern in Ireland and Sweden, of equal concern in the UK and Germany and hormones of more concern in Spain. Respondents in all countries agreed that fat or cholesterol in chicken was of least concern.

TABLE 5.
GROUPING OF CHICKEN CONCERNS WITHIN EACH COUNTRY
(A = highest, D = lowest)

Concern	Ireland	United Kingdom	Sweden	Germany	Spain	Italy
hormones	C	B	C	B	A	A
antibiotics	B	B	B	B	B	A
fat or cholesterol	D	C	D	C	C	B
bacteria/*Salmonella*	A	A	A	A	A	A

The results for concern about bacteria/*Salmonella* in chicken are shown in detail in Fig. 4. Some of the highest levels of concern were shown about bacteria/*Salmonella*; however, the level of concern was not consistent across countries. In both Ireland and Sweden 81% of consumers said that they were "very concerned" while, at the other end of the scale, only 48% of Italian consumers were "very concerned" on this issue.

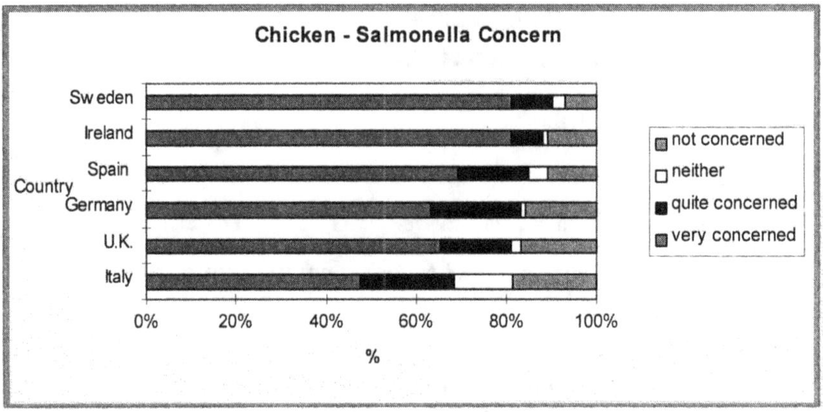

*Chi square = 257 ***, n = 2832*

FIG. 4. CONCERN ABOUT BACTERIA/*SALMONELLA* WHEN BUYING CHICKEN

Ranking Concerns Between Countries. For ease of presentation, the concerns were also ranked between countries. Table 6 shows the results for concerns relating to beef, pork and chicken. These rankings illustrate that, overall: (1) Spanish and Irish consumers are most concerned about the safety of meat, (2) British consumers are least concerned, and (3) Swedish, German and Italian consumers are intermediate in their concerns. However, consumers in Sweden, Germany and Italy are more concerned than consumers in most other countries about particular issues. The Swedes are more concerned about *Salmonella* in chicken, the Germans are more concerned (apart from the Irish) about BSE and the Italians are more concerned (apart from the Spanish) about fat in all three meats.

TABLE 6.
RANKING OF CONCERNS ABOUT MEATS ACROSS THE SIX COUNTRIES
(1 = highest, 6 = lowest)

(a) Beef

Concern	Ireland	United Kingdom	Sweden	Germany	Spain	Italy
hormones	2	6	5	4	1	3
antibiotics	2	6	4	3	1	5
fat or cholesterol	3	4	5	6	1	2
bacteria/ *Salmonella*	2	5	3	6	1	4
BSE	1	6	4	2	3	5

(b) Pork

Concern	Ireland	United Kingdom	Sweden	Germany	Spain	Italy
hormones	2	6	4	3	1	5
antibiotics	2	5	4	3	1	6
fat or cholesterol	2	4	5	6	1	2
bacteria/*Salmonella*	2	4	3	5	1	6

(c) Chicken

Concern	Ireland	United Kingdom	Sweden	Germany	Spain	Italy
hormones	2	6	5	4	1	3
antibiotics	1	6	3	4	2	5
fat or cholesterol	3	4	6	5	1	2
bacteria/*Salmonella*	2	4	1	4	3	6

Helpfulness of Factors in Assessing Safety When Buying Meat

Consumers were asked how helpful each of the following eight factors are in assessing the safety of the three meats: (1) what the animal was fed, (2) a brand or quality assurance label, (3) the name of the producer or farmer, (4) organic production (beef/pork only), (5) the country of origin, (6) the price, (7) freshness, and (8) free range production (chicken only). The extent to which this information is actually available to consumers varies both spatially and temporally. Table 7, for the combined data, summarises the results for the six countries. For the three meats, freshness, country of origin and the type of feed used were regarded as the most helpful safety indicators. Data on the range, for lowest to highest, show that the extent to which each factor is regarded as helpful varies considerably.

TABLE 7.
FACTORS PERCEIVED TO BE HELPFUL IN ASSESSING SAFETY — SIX COUNTRY AVERAGES

Factor	Proportion of consumers (%) saying factor is "very helpful"					
	Beef		Pork		Chicken	
	average	range	average	range	average	range
animal feed	61	(44-82)	56	(40-82)	59	(53-83)
quality label/brand	54	(40-70)	50	(38-66)	50	(35-65)
producer name	38	(23-66)	37	(22-59)	38	(22-61)
country of origin	67	(51-84)	56	(41-78)	53	(37-76)
freshness	78	(58-89)	81	(66-89)	81	(65-91)
organic production	46	(29-67)	45	(29-63)	-	
price	27	(10-39)	24	(13-36)	25	(16-34)
free range	-		-		62	(40-76)

For presentation of the detailed results by country the average scores for each helpfulness factor were calculated and the factors were then ranked within each country. Factors not statistically different are grouped together.

Beef. The within-country groups are shown in Table 8. Freshness is the most helpful factor in four of the six countries (Ireland, UK, Sweden and Spain) while, along with what the animal was fed, it is also the most helpful in Italy and is the second most helpful in Germany. What the animal was fed on and country of origin are the next most helpful factors across the countries. Type of feed is regarded as a very helpful indicator in Italy, and is in the second most helpful group in UK and Spain. Country of origin is most helpful in Germany, and is in the second most helpful group in Ireland, Sweden and Italy. A brand or quality label is in the second most helpful group in the UK and Italy. Organically produced is also in the second most helpful group in Italy. Price and the name of the producer are considered the least helpful factors in most countries.

TABLE 8.
HELPFULNESS OF FACTORS IN ASSESSING THE SAFETY OF BEEF WITHIN EACH COUNTRY
(A = most helpful, F = least helpful)

Factor	Ireland	United Kingdom	Sweden	Germany	Spain	Italy
What animal was fed on	C	B	D	C	B	A
Brand/quality assurance label	C	B	C	D	D	B
Name of producer	D	E	F	D	E	B
Organically produced	C	C	E	D	C	B
Country of origin	B	C	B	A	C	B
Price	E	D	F	E	E	C
Freshness	A	A	A	B	A	A

Pork. The within-country groups are shown in Table 9. Pork followed a somewhat similar pattern to beef with freshness being the most important factor in all of the countries. In Italy what the animal is fed is also grouped first with freshness. Organic production is among the second most helpful group in all countries except Sweden and what the animal is fed and country of origin are in the second most helpful group in four of the six. A quality label is in the second most helpful group for assessing the safety of pork in the UK, Ireland and Italy. As with beef the name of the producer and price are the least helpful factors.

Chicken. The within-country groups are shown in Table 10. Similar trends as for pork emerge in the case of chicken, with freshness being the most helpful factor in all six countries. Italy has animal feed as equally helpful as freshness. Free range is grouped in the second group (after freshness) in five countries with Sweden having it down the list in fifth place. What the chicken was fed is in the second group for the UK and Spain. For the UK, a brand or quality assurance label is also in the second most helpful group of factors while for Sweden country of origin is in this group. The name of the producer and price are the factors that are ranked lowest for assessing the safety of chicken across the six countries.

TABLE 9.
HELPFULNESS OF FACTORS IN ASSESSING THE SAFETY OF PORK WITHIN EACH COUNTRY
(A = most helpful, F = least helpful)

	Ireland	United Kingdom	Sweden	Germany	Spain	Italy
What animal was fed on	B	B	D	B	B	A
Brand/quality assurance label	B	B	C	C	C	B
Name of producer	C	D	F	C	D	B
Organically produced	B	B	E	B	B	B
Country of origin	B	C	B	B	C	B
Price	D	C	F	D	D	C
Freshness	A	A	A	A	A	A

TABLE 10.
HELPFULNESS OF FACTORS IN ASSESSING THE SAFETY OF CHICKEN WITHIN EACH COUNTRY
(A = most helpful, F = least helpful)

	Ireland	United Kingdom	Sweden	Germany	Spain	Italy
What chicken was fed on	C	B	D	C	B	A
Brand/quality assurance label	C	B	C	E	C	C
Name of producer	C	C	F	F	D	C
Country of origin	B	C	B	D	C	C
Price	D	C	F	G	D	D
Freshness	A	A	A	A	A	A
Free range	B	B	E	B	B	B

Helpfulness Scores Between Countries. The within-country rankings are shown in Table 11 for beef, pork and chicken. These rankings illustrate that for beef.

(1) In general, Irish consumers were more likely than consumers in other countries to find the various factors helpful in assessing beef quality at the time of purchase.
(2) The Italians were most likely to believe that information on the type of animal feed used is helpful.
(3) UK consumers were most likely to feel that price information is a helpful indicator.

TABLE 11.
HELPFULNESS OF FACTORS IN ASSESSING THE SAFETY OF MEATS ACROSS THE SIX COUNTRIES (RANKS)

(a) Beef

Factor	Ireland	United Kingdom	Sweden	Germany	Spain	Italy
What animal was fed on	2	5	6	4	2	1
Brand/quality assurance label	1	3	2	5	6	4
Name of producer	1	4	6	2	5	3
Organically produced	1	4	6	3	2	3
Country of origin	1	6	2	3	5	4
Price	2	1	5	6	4	3
Freshness	1	4	3	6	2	5

(b) Pork

Factor	Ireland	United Kingdom	Sweden	Germany	Spain	Italy
What animal was fed on	3	5	6	3	2	1
Brand/quality assurance label	2	3	1	5	6	4
Name of producer	1	4	5	3	6	2
Organically produced	1	2	5	3	4	6
Country of origin	2	5	1	3	6	4
Price	2	1	4	6	5	3
Freshness	3	1	2	6	4	5

(c) Chicken

Factor	Ireland	United Kingdom	Sweden	Germany	Spain	Italy
What chicken was fed on	4	5	6	3	2	1
Brand/quality assurance label	2	3	1	5	6	4
Name of producer	1	4	5	3	6	2
Country of origin	2	6	1	3	5	4
Price	3	1	6	5	4	2
Freshness	1	2	5	6	3	4
Free range	2	5	6	4	3	1

In the case of pork and chicken, Irish consumers, in general, were more likely than consumers in other countries to find the various factors helpful in assessing quality at the time of purchase. The Italians found information on feed very helpful while the Swedish consumers were more likely to find a quality label or information on the country of origin helpful. The UK consumers, as in the case of beef, were most likely to feel that price information is a helpful indicator. German consumers were more likely to find the name of the producer and the country of origin, and Spanish consumers the type of feed and freshness (except in the case of pork), more helpful than consumers in most other countries.

Who Consumers Most Trust When Looking for Information on Meat Safety

An open-ended question was used to ask respondents who they trust most when looking for information on the safety of meat. As many as three answers were recorded from each respondent. The five most-mentioned answers for each country are recorded in Table 12.

TABLE 12.
WHO, OR WHAT, CONSUMERS MOST TRUST FOR INFORMATION ON MEAT SAFETY
(1 = highest, 5 = lowest)

Ranking	Ireland	United Kingdom	Sweden	Germany	Spain	Italy
1	Butcher in the supermarket	Butcher in the supermarket	Media reports	Independent retailers/ butchers	Independent retailers/ butchers	Independent retailers/ butchers
2	Independent retailers/ butchers	Independent retailers/ butchers	Independent retailers/ butchers	Media reports	Butcher in the supermarket	Butcher in the supermarket
3	Media reports	Media reports	Butcher in the supermarket	Butcher in the supermarket	Government departments/ agencies	Media reports
4	Own opinion family and friends	Own opinion family and friends	Own opinion family and friends	Consumer groups	Own opinion family and friends	Government departments/ agencies
5	Government departments/ agencies	Government departments/ agencies	Government departments/ agencies	Own opinion family and friends	Media reports	Own opinion family and friends

Note 1: 30-40% of respondents in each country had no opinion when asked who they look to for information on the safety of their meat.

Note 2: Government departments/agencies include government, departments of agriculture, departments of health and food safety boards.

Note 3: Media reports include magazines, reports, radio reports, newspapers, food writers and television.

Butchers are the most trusted people throughout the six countries. In most countries, over 50% of mentions were of retail butchers. Media reports figured very highly in Sweden. They were ranked far higher than government departments/agencies. In all countries, except Spain, the media were ranked higher than government departments/agencies. In Germany, consumer groups were ranked fourth, the only country where they were mentioned and government departments/agencies did not figure in the first five mentions.

Attitude Statements

Respondents were asked for their attitudes towards a number of issues about food and meat. Their responses to three of these, dealing with buying local food, the country of origin of meat and confidence that the food that they are buying in the shops is safe, are shown in Table 13.

TABLE 13.
RANKING ATTITUDE STATEMENTS ACROSS COUNTRIES
(1 = highest, 6 = lowest)

Attitude	Ireland	United Kingdom	Sweden	Germany	Spain	Italy
I prefer to buy food which is produced locally	1	6	5	4	2	3
It is important that I know the country where the meat I buy has been produced	2	6	1	3	4	4
I am confident that the food in the shop is safe	4	6	1	5	2	3

The Irish consumers were ranked highest for their preference for buying food that is produced locally. When asked about the provision of information on the country of origin, the Swedish consumers were ranked highest, followed by the Irish and the German consumers. The Swedish, Spanish and Italian consumers have the most confidence that the food in their shops is safe. For each of these statements the United Kingdom consumers were ranked the lowest of the six countries.

The results show a strong preference among consumers for buying local foods and for wanting information on the country of origin of the meat they buy. This preference for local foods was strongest in Spain (77% agreeing strongly) and Ireland (79%) and weakest in the UK (43%) and Sweden (48%). The Swedish (81%) and Irish (78%) consumers were more likely to agree strongly that it is important to have information on the country of origin, while UK (42%) consumers were the least likely to agree. Some 33% of all those surveyed were not confident that the food in shops is safe. Sweden had the lowest lack of confidence (22%) and the UK the highest (41%).

YOUNG PEOPLE'S ATTITUDES TO MEAT

While two-thirds of those surveyed were eating more or the same amount of beef compared with a year previously, one-third have stopped or were eating less (Table 14). When asked whether eating beef meant increasing the risk of getting CJD, some 51% agreed (Fig. 5). This group was much more likely to have stopped eating beef or to be eating less beef than a year previously. On the other hand, young people who don't think about food and just eat what they are given were much less likely to have reduced or stopped eating beef. This key group of contented beef eaters represented about 28% of young people (Table 15).

TABLE 14.
AMOUNT OF BEEF EATEN NOW COMPARED WITH A YEAR PREVIOUSLY

Situation compared with last year	Proportion of sample (%)
eating more beef	17
eating same amount of beef	46
eating less beef	30
stopped eating beef	7

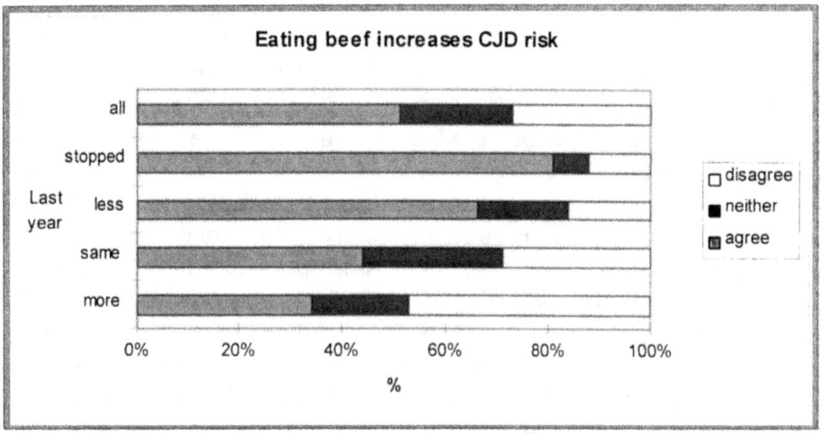

FIG. 5. VIEWS ON WHETHER EATING BEEF INCREASES RISK OF GETTING CJD

TABLE 15.
DECISION ON WHAT TYPE OF FOOD EATEN

Situation compared with last year	Response (%) to statement that "I don't think about food, I just eat what I am given"		
	Agree	Neither agree nor disagree	Disagree
Those eating more beef	46	18	36
Those eating same amount of beef	44	18	36
Those eating less beef	27	14	59
Those stopped eating beef	23	9	68
Average for all young people surveyed	38	16	46

With regard to the degree of confidence that adolescents have in what various companies, groups and organisations say about meat-related issues, the greatest confidence was in professionals such as doctors and scientists (Table 16). After these professionals, the next level of confidence was in Department of Health spokespersons, followed by a group including the Department of Agriculture and Food spokespersons, teachers, farmer representatives and food companies. Following these categories were the various media in which young people tended to have about the same degree of confidence. Finally, those in whom there was the least confidence in what is said about meat issues were politicians and elected representatives.

DISCUSSION AND CONCLUSIONS

Concerns

Bacteria/*Salmonella* was the issue of greatest concern in the case of chicken. For beef and pork, antibiotics and growth promoters were equally important concerns. BSE was also a major concern. As antibiotics in beef and growth promoters in pork are not an issue in reality, these results illustrate consumer confusion between real and low risk issues. The finding of consumer confusion is consistent with the findings for other studies in the last ten years (O'Neill *et al.* 1993). Although quality policies address the issues of antibiotics and growth promoters, consumers remain uncertain about these issues. Therefore, reducing this uncertainty is a key point for quality policy and illustrates the need to improve the information flow to consumers. In addition, understanding why concern about BSE varies between consumers in the different countries needs further study.

TABLE 16.
EXTENT OF CONFIDENCE IN STATEMENTS ON MEAT RELATED ISSUES

Group	Response (%) to question "how much confidence would you say you have in what the following have to say about meat related issues?"		
	Total or a great deal of confidence	Mixed reaction	Very little or no confidence
Doctors	72	19	10
Scientists	61	25	14
Dept. of Health spokespersons	54	29	17
Dept. of Agriculture and Food spokespersons	34	38	28
Teachers	32	44	25
Farmers representatives	28	39	33
Food-companies representatives	20	36	44
Newspaper articles	19	41	40
Food advertisers	19	25	56
TV programs	15	36	49
Radio programs	14	41	45
Magazine articles	12	40	48
Politicians and elected representatives	8	39	53

Note: the number surveyed in each category varied from 1242 to 1249

EU regulations forbid the use of growth hormones in beef animals and regular testing is undertaken. As the use of growth promoters in beef continues to be a major concern for consumers, clearly the increased and ongoing attention being paid to this issue by all quality policy instruments must be maintained. Similarly, there are limits on the levels of antibiotic residues permitted in pork. The ultimate objective must be to realise a situation where consumers can be assured that their beef is free from growth promoters, their pork is free from antibiotics (or that residues are below the specified limits) and that there is no confusion about these issues.

Nearly 40% of young Irish people were not too concerned about food risks and most of these were not reducing their beef consumption. On the other hand, about half of those interviewed believed that eating beef increases the risk of getting CJD and many of these were reducing consumption. This result highlights the difficulties facing the beef industry and points out the need to eliminate BSE. Only then can young, or other, consumers be expected to change their perceptions and consumption behaviour.

In the case of bacteria/*Salmonella*, the need for maintaining hygiene standards needs reiteration. Fresh meat handling techniques must be improved and carefully monitored to ensure that food poisoning risks for consumers are minimised.

The variation in level of concern on the various issues between countries is noteworthy. Overall, the Spanish were the most concerned about the safety of meat. They were ranked highest across the six countries on the issues of hormones and fat/cholesterol for the three meats. The Irish were the second most concerned while the UK consumers were the least concerned. The relatively low level of concern in the UK is an interesting find given the extent of media coverage of these issues during the year before the survey and despite BSE being a major issue for the UK.

Safety Indicators

Freshness is perceived to be the most helpful factor in assessing safety at the time of purchase for all three meats. Country of origin is regarded as the next most helpful factor. Ways of providing meaningful information on freshness should be considered for quality assurance schemes. Priority needs to be given when packing meat to ensuring that information on the freshness of the meat is clearly given. Date stamping is standard but perhaps further research on the consumer concept of freshness would identify other suitable ways of providing information on freshness. Consumers, particularly beef consumers in Sweden, Ireland and Germany, put a lot of emphasis on country of origin as a safety indicator. This suggests that consumers should be given this information for the meat they buy, particularly in the case of beef. Recent EU policy changes encourage this approach. The onus lies with industry in each country to ensure that the meat produced in its country is safe. Implementation of any scheme which assures safety is clearly difficult as any failures would destroy its credibility.

Of the other factors, free range was an important safety indicator in the case of chicken. What the animal is fed was perceived as being very helpful in assessing the safety of the three meats in Italy and to a lesser extent in other countries. Irish exporters could use the grass-fed beef image to advantage in this regard. Quality labels, while helpful (particularly in the UK and Sweden), did not top the agenda and this merits some debate. In Ireland's case, was it because quality labels and schemes are not long enough in existence or in widespread usage. Or was it because consumers don't understand what they mean or that the quality of information and/or the communication is poor? There is a need to provide consumers with information on schemes and labels and on what the labels mean.

The fact that meat was organically produced (for beef and pork) was not ranked as highly as a safety indicator as other factors. This was due probably to the low volume of organic meat produced rather than to any particular perception of the safety of this type of meat. For the three meats, information on price and name of producer were ranked the lowest.

Attitudes

There were differences in consumers' attitudes towards the origin of the meat. The Irish, Spanish, Italians and Germans said that they have a high preference for food that is produced locally. In these countries it would be more beneficial to have information on the region of production. This is less necessary in the case of Sweden and the United Kingdom. Confidence that food in shops is safe was not as high as it should be. The Swedes had the most confidence and the British the least. This is a little surprising in that the British also said that they are the least concerned about the safety of meat. There is a need for the food industry throughout the six countries to build on the confidence that does exist, using authentic information, thus reassuring consumers about food safety. Approaches that achieve this objective should be invested in.

Butchers were the most trusted people whether they are in the supermarket or are independent retailers. This strength should be built upon; removal of the butcher from counter service in the supermarket, as is the current trend, is likely to have a negative impact. The fact that the scientists and doctors were seen as the source of information that young people have most confidence in, is a positive outcome. The provision of objective information to consumers is essential and this result suggests that statements on food issues by agencies, such as a Food Safety Board, should highlight the fact when such statements are backed by scientific and medical evidence.

Consumption

Despite high levels of concern about bacteria/*Salmonella* in chicken, consumption has continued to increase. Clearly some concerns are impacting on meat consumption to a much greater degree than others. It must be concluded that the need for consumer safety assurance is greater for beef than for any other meat.

ACKNOWLEDGMENTS

Support from the Commission of the European Communities, Agriculture and Fisheries (FAIR) specific RTD programme, CT-95-0046 "Quality Policy and Consumer Behavior", and EU Structural Funds (European Regional Development Fund) is acknowledged. The first part of the paper reports on the work of the teams in six countries; the contribution of colleagues from the universities of Göttingen, Reading, Pisa, Madrid and Uppsala is equally acknowledged. The contributions of Michael Mannion and Seamus Rowe to analysis of the Irish and EU data are acknowledged. Particular thanks are due to Kristina Glitsch from Göttingen, and Spencer Henson from Reading. For the second part, on the survey of adolescents, the work presented is based on the research of Bridin McIntyre. Her contribution is also acknowledged.

REFERENCES

O'NEILL, F. and SHANAHAN, U. 1993. Dietary concerns of Irish consumers - second update. Socio Economic Research Series, No. 12, Teagasc.

STEENKAMP, J.B. 1989. Product Quality. An investigation into the concept and how it is perceived by consumers. Van Gorcum, Assen/Maastricht, The Netherlands.

VOSEN, T., MIKEL, W., MULVANEY, D. and JONES, R. 1992. A survey of consumer attitudes towards beef safety. Dairy, Food and Environmental Sanitation *12* (10) 621–624.

CHAPTER 3

EUROPEAN STRATEGIES FOR FOOD SAFETY CONTROL

PETER PRENDERGAST

Food and Veterinary Office
Consumer Policy and Consumer Health Protection
Directorate-General XXIV, European Commission
Trident House, Rock Hill
Blackrock, Co. Dublin, Ireland

ABSTRACT

From the perspective of the Food and Veterinary Office, which is part of Directorate General (DG) XXIV of the European Commission, an outline will be presented on the nature of the consumer confidence problem which has been developing over a number of years, giving a snapshot of consumer opinion in the European Union (EU) taken in Spring 1997. A picture will be presented of the changes in thinking and strategy within the Commission which have resulted in changes in its approach and the structure and responsibility of its services. Arising from this re-allocation of responsibilities, the Commission has adopted a new approach which is being implemented progressively. These developments will be described and comments made on some aspects. The Commission is considering the report of its Inspectorate General on its study and survey of food safety structures, strategies and techniques in the Member States and some selected third countries. This is designed to ensure that the EU approach takes account of any developments which could ensure the most effective system of food safety control. Areas will be identified which are suggested as necessary in the future and which will lead to possible future changes in strategy.

INTRODUCTION

Consumer policy within the European Commission started as a small part of the Environment Department but in recent times has become independent of all departments. Consumer Policy and Consumer Health Protection is now called Directorate General (DG) XXIV, and is assuming considerable importance since the Commission was faced with the fallout from the Bovine Spongiform Encephalopathy (BSE) crisis in cattle in the United Kingdom (UK). The Commission has moved a wide range of activities from other departments in the

Commission to DG XXIV and has made it responsible in the main for public safety in relation to food.

BACKGROUND

A series of factors have influenced the shaping of consumer attitudes in Europe and European consumer doubts about the safety (wholesomeness) of food products. Quite clearly there is a widespread awareness of the Common Agricultural Policy (CAP) and the belief that the main aim of the European Union (EU) and of governments is to keep farmers happy. This perception has been supported by examples of many actions to appease the agriculture lobby and by the apparent over-riding concern regarding a farming backlash in a number of countries. For example, in France when the farmers get upset about some issue they take direct action like blocking roads and breaking shop windows and the government inevitably settles with them. This confirms the consumers' observation that there is a huge interest and support in favour of farming and the farming community.

There is a mistrust of government and public authorities by many European citizens. For example, after the dramatic accident at Chernobyl, the Chernobyl radioactive cloud was reported to have crossed Europe until it got to the bridge in Strasbourg, dividing Germany from France. According to the French government of the time, the cloud stopped and went out over Belgium and Holland to Scotland! It took the French consumers about three months to realise that, at worst, the Government had lied to them and, at best, they had been economical with the truth. A similar kind of thing happened in relation to blood, arising from the AIDS crisis. In France, Germany and Italy huge scandals occurred in relation to blood, with the public authorities failing, despite apparently having knowledge, to take the kind of action that would protect people.

Then there is the observation of intensification of agricultural production, partly arising from CAP, which puts a big emphasis on volume output and the associated heavy use of fertilisers, antibiotics and pesticides. People are aware that high volume production leads to concerns about animal welfare. They are aware that intensive production increases the possibility of bacterial contamination of food. There is the illegal use of hormones and the apparent disregard for the law in some countries by small numbers of farmers. It is a criminal offence to use these substances in Europe but, despite that, in all countries there has been constant evidence, through the media, of serious breaches of that law. In Belgium, there was a particular crisis because one of the chief veterinary inspectors was assassinated. This caused huge distress and the daily reports in Belgian newspapers about the "hormone mafia" contribute to a very negative consumer view.

There have been a number of European consumer studies, professionally carried out and disseminated very widely, which have studied issues such as clenbuterol and hormonal growth promoters in beef. One particular study found that 23% of all beef liver at the point of sale to the consumer in Belgium contained clenbuterol, being, almost a "clenbuterol cocktail" rather than liver; the figure for Spain was 36% clenbuterol positive. Seven percent of entrecote steak in Belgium contained residues of hormonal growth promoters. Another study, on the occurrence of antibiotic residues in pork, carried out across the EU indicated the occurrence of residue-positive product in a number of member states. A study on the microbiological status of chicken meat at point of sale found that about 60% of all chicken in Europe was contaminated with either *Salmonella* or *Campylobacter*. Only one country appeared to have no *Salmonella* on chicken and that was Sweden; the *Campylobacter* level was not studied there. All of this information is feeding into the public's mind, shaping attitudes and concerns.

Then there is the whole area of "green" issues, controversy about veal crates and about overcrowding of chickens in poultry production units. While unrelated to food production, there is the very big controversy in some of the European member states about vivisection and about testing cosmetics on animals. People react very negatively to this picture of a lack of concern for animals and for animal welfare.

Returning to food issues, there have been some major scandals such as the wine scandal in Austria when anti-freeze was put into the wine. A few years later this also happened in Italy, with the Veneto wines which had to be taken off the supermarket shelves in the UK. Then there was the Spanish olive oil calamity where 36 people died as a result of using contaminated oil.

With the BSE outbreak, beef took the hit for all food. If it had been chicken, it would probably have suffered the same kind of consequences, given the background and given the negative feeling that people had developed. In relation to the BSE crisis, a very striking fact for most consumers which they could not understand was why those making the major decisions at Community level were fifteen veterinarians.

CONSUMER CONCERNS

Against this background of European consumer doubts about the safety of food, in February 1997 the Commission examined the situation in all fifteen member states. To get a measure of their real feelings, people were asked how worried they were about a whole variety of things, for example, medicines, cosmetics, toys, food, electrical appliances, public transport, cars, aeroplanes, restaurants, etc. The results of the survey showed that 68% of people were particularly concerned about the safety of food, 67% about the safety of medicines, and the level of concern in relation to other products and services was 38% (cleaning products), 33% (electrical appliances), 30% (public transport), 30% (toys), 29% (cars), 27% (aeroplanes), 26% (public places), 26% (cosmetics), 21% (restaurants), 20% (sports events) and 13% (hotels). Table 1 gives a breakdown of these figures by country.

The spectacular concern about food safety is notable. The expectation was that medicines would stand out on top because they are considered by public authorities to be unsafe in normal use, quite different from the traditional perception in relation to other products which were generally regarded as safe in normal use. That is why medicines have been subject to pre-marketing control, clinical testing, monitoring, etc. It appears now that in consumers' eyes food has managed to reach the same level of concern.

Table 1 shows the variation in concern about food safety between countries. This ranges from a high of 90% of French people identifying food as a problem, down to a low in Finland of 40%. With the EU average being at 68%, Ireland at 55% and the UK at 54% are below average in the scale of concern about food safety. The difference between member states is interesting particularly for Germany, which might have been expected to be at the top but which was close to the EU average. The biggest concern was in France, Luxembourg, Denmark, Sweden, Greece and Belgium.

EUROPEAN COMMISSION RESPONSE

That is the background against which the institutions of the EU have been reappraising how best to handle the issue of food safety. When the BSE crisis exploded after the UK House of Commons' statement of 20th March 1996, there was a calamitous reaction across Europe with very serious consequences for large sections of the food industry. Measures were taken to ring-fence the problem and a world ban on the export of British beef followed. The European Parliament used its new powers to establish an enquiry into what went wrong and produced a hard hitting report which was critical of many elements, including the Commission, the Member States and industry for failing to act. It established a BSE crisis committee to monitor how well its recommendations have been taken on board and its plenary session in November 1997 is to decide whether to censure the Commission or take some other action. Many of its recommendations have been acted upon.

Accordingly a new strategy has emerged at EU level to handle food issues:

1. A decision was taken to reorganise the Commission's own services so that control, inspection and monitoring activities would be separated from the law making and market management (agricultural policy) functions.

TABLE 1.

SURVEY OF EUROPEAN CONSUMERS IN FEBRUARY 1997 — REPLIES (%) TO THE QUESTION "WHICH OF THE FOLLOWING DO YOU FEEL PARTICULARLY CONCERNED ABOUT, AS REGARDS THE SAFETY OF PRODUCTS AND SERVICES FOR CONSUMERS?"

COUNTRY	B	DK	D west	D Total	D east	GR	E	F	IRL	I	L	NL	A	P	FIN	S	UK	EU 15
Medicines	75.4	84.7	58.6	59.2	61.3	75.9	59.9	88.5	58.4	63.5	71.0	86.5	49.9	52.8	42.2	96.6	60.7	67.3
Cosmetic products	28.9	27.2	28.3	27.6	25.0	43.8	14.5	39.7	20.5	20.0	34.6	25.1	20.3	12.5	22.4	30.9	21.3	25.6
Toys	39.5	39.8	11.7	11.9	12.8	21.9	25.2	51.6	34.5	12.0	37.2	47.8	9.6	19.2	26.3	61.9	50.5	29.9
Food	76.8	82.3	66.9	66.6	65.6	78.1	68.4	90.7	55.4	61.3	86.8	72.6	52.9	51.0	39.3	80.1	54.1	67.9
Electrical appliances	57.6	53.7	11.2	10.5	7.6	14.0	18.7	66.5	30.4	19.3	71.2	57.6	11.3	32.2	53.7	69.6	41.1	32.7
Cars	52.2	47.9	8.5	8.5	8.6	22.5	25.1	66.8	21.7	15.3	62.3	47.9	8.5	24.9	5.2	55.8	28.6	28.7
Public places (shops, theatres, cinema, etc.)	44.9	25.8	11.7	12.9	17.6	15.0	24.1	57.8	20.4	19.0	59.7	31.7	10.0	23.4	6.2	34.9	21.8	25.8
Hotels	23.9	17.2	4.3	4.4	4.5	10.5	10.7	28.6	14.0	6.7	31.4	16.2	5.1	8.2	4.8	29.4	14.0	12.7
Sports events	25.1	19.1	11.8	13.5	20.1	15.7	21.1	33.6	21.4	20.3	36.9	19.8	7.9	15.1	5.5	30.7	17.8	20.1
Cleaning products	46.4	63.4	32.3	31.4	27.8	37.2	25.3	65.2	35.2	21.4	61.1	51.0	35.8	22.0	29.0	57.8	39.9	37.9
Public transport	38.1	42.5	10.0	11.6	17.6	23.1	28.2	55.0	21.4	29.3	53.1	41.9	14.3	30.0	6.8	52.1	31.6	30.1
Planes	27.6	37.9	26.1	26.8	29.3	21.3	13.5	41.1	18.9	24.6	40.6	39.0	17.4	7.4	14.9	63.3	21.5	26.8
Restaurants	37.4	20.6	8.3	8.3	8.3	20.6	16.7	48.6	20.5	13.1	55.7	22.8	8.2	19.5	6.9	35.0	20.8	20.9
None	5.1	1.2	10.7	9.9	6.8	4.1	10.6	0.6	13.6	5.9	2.9	2.1	13.3	18.3	10.6	0.1	11.8	7.6
Don't know	2.9	0.8	5.5	5.4	4.9	1.5	2.7	0.6	3.9	3.2	3.5	1.2	5.4	12.6	5.3	0.7	2.0	3.2

Adapted from "Eurobarometer 47.0" - February 1997

2. This has also happened with the security of scientific advice; because scientific advice is very important in the management of food problems which emerge, scientific advice should be located in DG XXIV under the consumer umbrella. In addition, strenuous efforts should be made to ensure the independence of scientific advice. The only hope and real guarantee of the independence of scientific advice, is widespread transparency. If the information being sought from scientists is published and open to scrutiny by their peers, there is a much better chance of securing unbiased advice. The scientists involved should not be represented on the scientific committees but should belong to the universities or research institutions in the appropriate areas of research.

3. A specialist risk assessment unit has been established to try to assess the risks to safety, to manage those risks and to communicate about the risks.

All these functions have been transferred to DG XXIV, which has responsibility for consumer policy, and processes are in hand to ensure that all these elements work effectively. The Food and Veterinary Office (FVO) is being established and is charged with inspecting and monitoring how the Member States manage food safety. In addition, the FVO is responsible for ensuring that all third countries meet the standards needed in the EU for any food they supply to this market.

The Commission established a special group of Commissioners, under the Presidency of the Commission President, to meet regularly and consider any aspects of food safety which arise. An interservice committee of key DGs, under the chairmanship of DG XXIV, has been set up to co-ordinate action. The Inspectorate General of the Commission was assigned to study how food safety was managed in all the Member States and selected third countries, such as the U.S.A., New Zealand and Canada and has reported recently. The Inspector General believes that the EU strategy outlined above is correct but needs to be developed further.

These are the elements which have emerged to provide the new strategy to manage food safety issues.

1. Monitoring to be carried out by agencies independent of industry.
2. Independent scientific advice.
3. Transparency — public availability of results and opinions, so that consumers, by being exposed to information, will eventually be in a position to do their own risk assessment.
4. Building up inspection resources and expertise in the FVO entrusted with ensuring that each national authority implements the European food laws.

5. Auditing approach — where relevant, the FVO will formally audit the safety control systems of all the member states and 270 third countries, who export food to the EU.
6. Real attempts to assess and manage risk.
7. Change product liability law to include primary food production; a legislative proposal has been produced by the Commission and it is expected that within two years product liability will cover the total primary food sector, just as it does every other sector.
8. Change sectoral laws to raise standards; food laws must be updated and improved.
9. Traceability of food, which has already been put in legislative form in relation to bovine meat and which will increasingly extend across the range of food.
10. Control from stable or field to table; control across the whole food chain, requiring new controls (not just veterinary) which will yield benefits and dividends in terms of safety.

By far the most important element in the whole mix of actions is the move towards increased transparency. The lack of transparency has contributed greatly to keeping consumers in ignorance, dependent on public authorities and the media for knowledge. When consumers get to mistrust the agriculture/food industry and the public agencies, the dramatic vulnerability of the whole food chain to scares and crises is profound.

THE FUTURE

It is important that work is carried out from the most credible base possible. The citizens of Europe were asked who they thought would be likely to tell the truth about the quality of food. The consumer organisations were not included because research over the years has shown that they have credibility. What emerged from this study was that the winners were scientists (36%), followed by teachers (33%), radio and television (22%) the press (21%), government agencies (7%) and the European Commission (11%). The European Commission is not at or near the top nor is it a good base from which to start, but it is the only base from which some credibility can come. The European Commission is not starting ahead of the posse, rather it is starting well behind the starting line and it is quite important for people to realise that. The kind of atmosphere and the kind of attitude that exists now in Europe on food safety is reflecting itself in the national policies of each of the individual member states. In this climate, the single market for food will come under immense pressure and, if that happens, it will have major consequences for every country in the European

Union. The idea of having a single market was painstakingly built up, but if the concerns about food are reflected in the populations, then the national governments will tend, and in some instances it will suit them economically, to try to re-nationalise more and more of the food policies. So what is at stake effectively in not addressing or handling the food safety issue properly, is the ability of all fifteen countries to trade freely in foodstuffs across frontiers in the EU.

If the FVO can get the support of the National Governments and other EU institutions to achieve its objectives, then significant improvement will be possible. The FVO can contribute to ensuring better food production, distribution and consumption. It can develop consumer knowledge, so that they can better assess the risks they face and accordingly bring an improvement to the environment within which the whole business operates in future. It will not be easy but it is probably the only realistic way forward.

CHAPTER 4

FOOD SAFETY – THE RETAILERS' PERSPECTIVE

W. PATERSON

Tesco, Ireland
Marine Road
Dunlaoghaire, Co Dublin, Ireland

ABSTRACT

Who has responsibility for ensuring food safety? This paper demonstrates how Tesco, as a major food retailer, approaches its responsibilities in the provision of safe, wholesome and nutritious foods to its customers. Tesco's commitment to Food Safety begins with growers and processors, extends through its supply chain and stores, to finally embrace the customer. Safety and quality is established at the outset by its team of Food Technologists working in close partnership with suppliers. In this the key element is the use of appropriate Quality Management Systems based on a detailed Hazard Analysis Critical Control Point (HACCP) review of processes.

As food enters the distribution system, Quality Assurance teams monitor incoming deliveries to ensure that they achieve agreed specifications with regard to quality, appearance and temperature. In the stores, training ensures that staff handle food in a safe manner. For example, staff who handle unwrapped food must pass a Food Safety examination. Store operations are designed using the principles of HACCP and reviewed by a team of Trading Law Managers, who verify that standards are being achieved and may carry out internal audits. Tesco recognises its role in keeping consumers informed about food safety. For example, a recently issued leaflet, "Food Safety — Everyone's Concern", clearly explains the steps Tesco takes to ensure product safety, and outlines the role of the consumer in maintaining product safety.

Although Food Safety is frequently defined as primarily a microbiological issue, customers may not perceive it as such. To many of them, food safety has a broader meaning, encompassing such areas as chemical or pesticide residues, growing conditions and genetic modification. This wider interpretation increases the challenges in providing clear customer information on this fundamental area which confronts everybody.

INTRODUCTION

This paper deals mainly with Tesco's approach to food safety in the UK, not all of which is currently in operation in Ireland. While it does not specifically deal with food science, the integration of this subject within the companies overall approach to food safety will be clearly demonstrated. The Tesco approach to safety will be considered under four headings: (1) Product management with suppliers, (2) Management of the supply chain, (3) In-store management and training, and (4) The customer perspective.

PRODUCT MANAGEMENT WITH SUPPLIERS

A key element in Tesco's approach to food safety is the involvement of its suppliers in ensuring that products meet the standards required by Tesco. This includes the work involved in building up relationships with suppliers. Tesco has more than fifty food technologists working with suppliers on a world wide basis. This work with suppliers draws heavily on two basic documents: (a) the Legal Compliance and Quality Management Systems manual, and (b) the General Guidance on Food Hygiene Requirements. These make it possible to clarify and emphasise supplier responsibility for legal compliance and the management of their own business. The majority of suppliers and the majority of businesses now fully understand the general guidelines on hygiene, and understand the targets they should aspire to, and the standards they must achieve.

Legal Compliance

Every Tesco brand product must have been subject to a complete and fully documented hazard analysis. If this process has not been completed, and full documentation is not available, the item will not be a Tesco brand product. Every supplier must have a quality management system in place, and that quality management system must be appropriate to the size of their business. A business employing 500 people may have a system which encompasses 20 or 30 files of material, whereas, for a small cheese maker employing five people, one file including the basic systems is appropriate. There must be complete traceability from the raw materials going into the process, right through the process, to the finished product and onto the store shelves. Suppliers must review their operations to ensure they have appropriate management, and apply adequate internal audit systems, to ensure that their business is running effectively. They must have an effective product recall system in place. Tesco does not insist on an ISO accredited BS standard, in that a good quality management system is considered an effective tool.

Food Hygiene

This breaks down into two key areas. The design and construction of premises must be correct for the product flow and the people working in the area. Floor construction and wall finishes must be appropriate and should be sealed and cleanable. The provision of services into the building and to the process areas must be considered. Detailed guidelines on equipment design, fitness for use, ease of cleaning, and food contact surfaces are provided.

Staff and personnel hygiene are considered in detail, including protective clothing, policies on the wearing of jewellery, etc. Particular attention is paid to the function and nature of staff facilities. As well as these two key elements, many other specific codes of practice, such as for high care products or canned products, are in place.

Some other key factors need to be highlighted. A food technologist must approve each facility that produces a Tesco brand product. Food technologists decide which product can be sourced from each facility. Each production unit is subject to re-audit within an agreed schedule, derived after a risk assessment, reviewing safety, legal and quality risks. Re-audit could be every six months to a year, as dictated by the risk assessment and Tesco's knowledge of each supply base. Each Tesco brand product must have a product specification, detailing microbiological and chemical standards, and the appropriate shelf life. The product must retain microbiological quality under normal storage conditions and remain organoleptically acceptable to the end of its shelf life. Routine surveillance of these parameters is carried out on products from the store.

Lastly, and very importantly customer feed-back, queries and complaints are closely monitored, and subject to trend analyses. The data obtained is reviewed to identify and resolve possible product problems.

MANAGEMENT OF THE SUPPLY CHAIN

Tesco depots handling chilled and frozen foods normally have a team of between five and seven quality assurance officers, whose main role is to ensure that the quality of these fresh food products is appropriate. They also monitor temperature regimes within the depots, to ensure a totally integrated and unbroken quality supply chain. These quality officers also make sure that handling and stacking procedures are correct to avoid product damage leading to a food safety risk.

IN STORE MANAGEMENT AND TRAINING

Appropriate staff training is the cornerstone of in-store food safety, and can be broken down into three areas.

Basic Food Hygiene and Personal Safety

Food safety courses and certification are provided for any member of the staff who handles unwrapped food. Staff working in such areas as the delicatessen counter or the fish counter must have a food safety certificate. This policy is backed up by detailed departmental training manuals containing comprehensive details on the correct way to cut different types of cheese, the methods and precautions in handling and filleting of fish, etc.

Training Manuals

Detailed training manuals have been developed for Tesco coffee shops, which cater to customers or the 160,000 Tesco employees who have to be fed every day. Store operations are based on a risk management review of procedures and systems using HACCP principles. For example, risk management has been applied to delicatessen counter operations. This process is very similar to a standard HACCP assessment. The area of operation is examined, and risks are identified. These determine the control measures that must be put into place. Departmental guides are available for every department so that operational procedures and training documents are available to ensure that staff are given the information they need to do their job correctly.

Legal Responsibilities

Law guides are provided to store management teams so that they know their legal responsibilities in delivering what the customer needs. For example, there is an information booklet on managing legal compliance which demonstrates everything that needs to be done to ensure legal compliance. Booklets are also available in such areas as food safety, health and safety, and pricing.

INTERNAL SYSTEMS AUDITS

As well as the above internal audits, retail management teams also carry out regular assessments, auditing in-house systems to make sure that training procedures are effective and appropriate. Additional independent internal audits are carried out by the training law managers, who are trained environmental health officers, working for Tesco. They report to the store managers who are required to take appropriate action. Other external audits by environmental health officers, training standards officers, etc. supply additional information. Finally, there are in effect, nine million other "external audits" carried out every week by customers who come into the stores, look at the products and systems and either buy or do not buy.

CUSTOMER PERSPECTIVE

This can be reviewed under two headings, firstly in terms of the information the company provides to customers on food safety; and secondly as the customer's perspective of food safety, or what they perceive food safety to be.

Customer Information

The key vehicle for providing information to consumers is the product. A Tesco brand product normally carries date codes, as well as usage and appropriate storage instructions. For example, these indicate if the product should be frozen, and for how long. A fresh product will provide the consumers with appropriate and detailed cooking instructions. These instructions may be the final safety reference that Tesco products have. Tesco have teams of people who work on new products to develop detailed instructions to ensure proper cooking and the achievement of adequate core temperatures across the range of microwave, frying or oven cooking.

Customer information leaflets form an important aspect. A recently published customer information leaflet outlined how "Food Safety Is Everyone's Concern". It indicates what Tesco does as a company to ensure food safety, and explains what customers must do to ensure their own safety. Information is provided on date codes, the differences between terms like "display by", "use by", "best before", and on those foods which are not currently date coded. It talks about customers' responsibilities in getting food from the shop to the home in a safe manner, in terms of correct packing of products and limiting journey times. Customers are also advised on the safe use of the refrigerator to avoid cross contamination between raw and cooked foods. Information on safe use of the freezer includes the "star" coding, storage of prefrozen products, and guidance on freezing and refreezing of foods. Detailed advice is provided on safe practice in heating and re-heating of food, and those foods which need special care. Overall kitchen hygiene — air drying of dishes, drying hands on separate towels, washing hands before and after handling raw foods, is reviewed within a format which presents information in a simple, effective manner which customers can easily understand.

Customer Perspective of Food Safety

What do consumers perceive as food safety? Sometimes questions are asked which are not simply in terms of "is it safe". For instance, Tesco may be asked if it is safe to drink milk containing dioxins. There is no simple answer to such a question. A microbiologist would consider food safety in terms of the absence of pathogens such as *Salmonella, E. coli* or *Campylobacter*. However, customers think of food safety in much broader terms, which include two different aspects:

(1) food safety and (2) food integrity, i.e., wholesomeness. In these terms "is it safe to eat" is much more complex. Retailers now need to be considering questions in relation to pesticides as an aspect of food integrity. Customers are asking: "what has been used to grow this product", "what is actually on our apples" or "what is on our sugar beet?" Customers now view genetic modification of foods, whether soya, corn, or other products, as a safety issue. Other concerns include the use of hormones in meat production and the whole area of the welfare and treatment of animals before finally arriving at the table. Environmental issues may also be involved. They are interested in the environmental impact of tiger prawn farming in Malaysia and the effects of slurry spreading on farm land and water courses. As well as such effects on the environment, customers are becoming more and more interested in the welfare of the food producers. Are the people who harvest those crops, whether in East Anglia or in China, being paid an appropriate rate?

The responsibility for providing appropriate customer information rests with the scientists, government bodies, retailers and the media — everybody has a part to play. A great deal has been said about who the customers can and cannot trust. Can they trust scientists, the government, or others agencies? More and more of their trust is now being placed in the retailer. Customers are asking Tesco more and more questions about food, particularly in relation to quality and safety. They are learning to trust retailers more and more in such aspects. For their part, retailers will have to justify that trust and respond to customers honestly by providing the correct information.

CHAPTER 5

FOOD SAFETY RESEARCH: DISSEMINATING THE RESULTS IN EUROPE AND IRELAND

T. R. GORMLEY and K. BRENNAN

Teagasc, The National Food Centre
Dunsinea, Castleknock
Dublin 15, Ireland

ABSTRACT

A rapid transfer of research results from researcher to end-user is of paramount importance for the utilisation of the data and for generating innovation. In the case of food safety research results, the need is even more pressing as consumer health may be the issue. FLAIR-FLOW EUROPE and IRL-FLOW are two ongoing (the former trans-Europe and the latter in Ireland) dissemination projects charged with the diffusion of results (including those on food safety) from European and national food R & D programmes to the food industry, health professionals and other end-users. The operating procedure and output of the two dissemination projects is described and titles of 45 recently completed and ongoing food safety research projects which are supported by European and national funds are listed.

INTRODUCTION

Reaching end users with results of research and development (R & D) is always a major challenge. There is often an imbalance between the amount of money spent on carrying out R & D, and that spent (relatively little) on ensuring effective and adequate dissemination of the results to end-users. In carrying out research there are five main steps: (1) planning the project, (2) seeking funding, (3) doing the research, (4) disseminating the results, (5) seeking exploitation and end use. Of the five, the last two are by far the most difficult and are often neglected by scientists as they finish one project and move on eagerly to a new one.

This paper describes two dissemination projects which have been established to address the above issue. The first is FLAIR-FLOW EUROPE (F-FE) (Anon. 1994; Gormley 1992, 1994, 1996a) which is a series of sequential projects (F-FE I 1991-1993; F-FE II 1994-1996; F-FE III 1997-2000) charged with the dissemination of food research results from European Union (EU) programmes, and notably from the FLAIR (Food-Linked Agro-Industrial Research), AAIR (Agriculture and Agro-Industry Research) and FAIR (Agriculture and Fisheries Research) programmes of Directorates General (DsG) XII and XIV. The information is disseminated to the food industry, health professionals and consumer groups in the 15 EU countries and in Norway, Iceland and Switzerland.

The second dissemination project (termed IRL-FLOW for convenience) is ongoing in Ireland only, and is disseminating results from the so-called Non-Commissioned Food Research Programme (Brennan 1997 a,b). This programme is part-funded by grant aid under the Food Sub Programme of the Operational Programme of Industrial Development which is administered by the Irish Department of Agriculture and Food and supported by national and EU funds (i.e. Structural Funds).

Both the EU Fourth Framework and the Non-Commissioned Food Research Programmes contain a number of research projects on food safety and the results are being disseminated by the FLAIR-FLOW EUROPE and IRL-FLOW projects, respectively. Details of the operating procedures of the two dissemination projects are given together with their output and the titles of the research projects on food safety.

FLAIR-FLOW EUROPE

Objectives and Operation

FLAIR-FLOW EUROPE III (1997-2000), II (1994-1996) and I (1991-1993) are sequential projects with FLAIR-FLOW III being built on the strengths of II and I. The aim of FLAIR-FLOW III is to disseminate the food research results emanating from the ongoing EU FAIR programme, and also some carry-over results from the now-completed AAIR and FLAIR programmes. FLAIR-FLOW is funded by the EU FAIR (DG XII) and INNOVATION (DG XIII) programmes. Many of the results are from research projects on food safety. Experience from the FLAIR-FLOW II project indicated that the structure embracing national dissemination networks (and network leaders) in each of the 18 participating countries was highly effective. The dissemination procedures used, i.e. user-friendly 1-page technical documents, their reproduction in trade journals, focused workshops [including RETUER (ready-to-use-European research) workshops], the internet, and other routes, were very fruitful (Fig. 1) and will be repeated, with upgrading, in FLAIR-FLOW III. In effect, FLAIR-FLOW is a 'matchmaker' and when end-users require more information they fax or e-mail the researcher named on the end of the 1-page technical document thus establishing a person to person link. The objectives of FLAIR-FLOW III are:

- To reach food SMEs (small to medium sized enterprises), health professionals and other end-users in 18 European countries (15 EU countries with Norway, Iceland and Switzerland) with the results from EU sponsored food research programmes (including food safety R & D) in user-friendly form; this will include the identification of new dissemination procedures.

- To extract the more vital/strategic results, including those on food safety, from the FAIR/AAIR programmes for end-users. This will embrace the preparation of manuals by consultants (separate mini contracts awarded by the EU Commission).

- To obtain feedback from food SMEs as to the usefulness and uptake of the RTD information coming from European food research. This activity will include the formation of a platform of food SMEs.

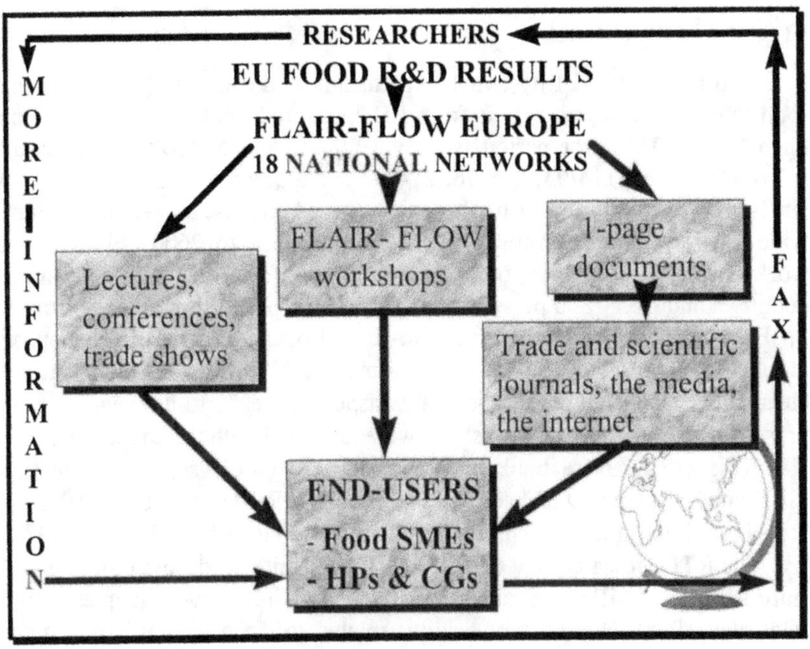

FIG. 1. *FLAIR FLOW*: ROUTES FOR INFORMATION TRANSFER
SMEs = Small to medium enterprises
HPs = Health professionals
CGs = Consumer groups

- To promote innovation in the European food industry through the diffusion of RTD results to food SMEs and by bringing the actors together, i.e. the technology providers (researchers) on the one hand, and the technology users (food SMEs and other end-users) on the other.

- To quantify output and feedback in the FLAIR-FLOW III project.

- To form dynamic interactive links with the network of European INNOVATION Relay Centres, with the network of FAIR Focal Points, with the European Union of Consumers, and with other relevant groups.

From these objectives, it is clear that FLAIR-FLOW III is both a dissemination and a research project. The latter refers to identifying new dissemination routes, the pinpointing of food SME R & D requirements, the assessment (by SMEs) of the quality and usefulness of the FLAIR-FLOW III project output, and the identification of ways to encourage food SMEs to use the results from EU-sponsored food research, i.e. the project also promotes and encourages innovation in this important industry sector.

FLAIR-FLOW output

Two hundred and fifty two 1-page technical documents (many relating to food safety) on research results from EU sponsored food research programmes have been issued in the period January 1991 to October 1997 and are collated in booklets F-FE 114/93, 236/96, 274/97 and also on the FLAIR-FLOW web site http://www.exp.ie/flair.html. Articles based on these are published Europe-wide in trade and scientific journals and amount to 2600. FLAIR-FLOW workshops (147 in number; 66 of them on food safety) have been held in the 18 countries and over 7800 persons attended, a high proportion of them from food SMEs. Four pilot 'RETUER' (ready-to-use European research) workshops were targeted at small food SMEs, and 'near-market' results on food equipment cleanability and on the safety and quality aspects of ready-to-use vegetables were presented. Three seafood workshops were also held with the cooperation of DG XIV (Fisheries) and a booklet (F-FE 199/96) on EU seafood projects was distributed. The output and activities of the FLAIR-FLOW I, II and III projects are highlighted in three technical circulars (Gormley 1993, 1996b, 1997).

The RTD (research and technical development) needs and opinions of 809 European food SMEs were canvassed in 1994 via interviews and questionnaires (Gormley 1995). One of the questions related to the percentage of companies making 'large' investments in five areas with the following results: new equipment (82%); processes (64%); hygiene (51%); safety (39%); quality (65%). Hygiene and safety were split as two separate questions and the percentage of companies making large investments in safety was surprisingly small. This begs the question would the percentage have been much larger in 1997 (i.e. three years after the survey) when, presumably, companies were more aware of the importance of food safety due to the BSE and *E. coli* outbreaks. In a second survey (Gormley 1995) 105 companies were interviewed as to their research, development and technology needs. The percentage responses were as follows: food quality (20%); product development/improvement/modification (18%); technology (13%); food safety (8%); other areas (41%). Again the percentage of companies citing food safety as a major RTD need was small.

EU Sponsored Food Safety Research

The food safety projects in the EU FLAIR, AAIR and FAIR programmes are given in Table 1. All of the projects in the FLAIR programme are completed as are most in the AAIR programme, while those in the FAIR programme are ongoing.

TABLE 1.
FOOD SAFETY RESEARCH PROJECTS[1] IN THE EU FLAIR, AAIR AND FAIR PROGRAMMES

FLAIR programme

- Predictive modelling of bacteria
- Controlling poultry pathogens
- HACCP and hurdle technology
- Toxicology and residues
- Limited shelf life products
- MAP of meat products
- Natural antimicrobials
- Food plant sanitation
- Raw milk vs cheese safety

AAIR programme

- Spoilage yeasts in foods and beverages
- Human cell lines for safety evaluation of foods
- Transgenic food crops
- Safety of ready-to-eat foods
- Safety of foods processed by sous-vide
- Air sterility in food factories
- Physiology of food poisoning microorganisms
- Risk to health from natural food toxicants
- Safety of biotech. processes and products

FAIR programme

- Verotoxigenic *E. coli*
- Safety criteria for minimally processed foods
- Decontamination of meat and meat products
- Microbiological quality of mineral water
- Novel antimicrobial systems
- Rapid detection of mould contamination
- Nisin & biopreservative combinations
- Biomarkers versus deleterious diets
- Frozen food safety in the distribution chain
- Immunochemical test methods
- Molecular imprint - based technology

[1] Most are abbreviated titles

The projects (Table 1) collectively represent a major commitment by the EU to food safety research, and 1-page documents will be issued on the FAIR projects as the results become available over the next three years. The FAIR and AAIR food safety projects have been the subject of 66 FLAIR-FLOW workshops (Europe-wide) to date.

Information on FLAIR-FLOW EUROPE

Contact Ronan Gormley (FLAIR-FLOW Project Leader), Gerry Downey or Patricia Moriarty at Teagasc, The National Food Centre, Dunsinea, Castleknock, Dublin 15, Ireland. Tel + 353-1-8059500; Fax: + 353-1-8059550; e-mail: p.moriarty@nfc.teagasc.ie or visit the FLAIR-FLOW web site http://www.exp.ie/flair.html.

IRL-FLOW

Objectives and Operation

The IRL-FLOW dissemination project commenced in April 1996 and will terminate in December 1999. It is based on the FLAIR-FLOW model but with some modifications. It operates in Ireland only and has the overall objective of disseminating and promoting the results from the Non-Commissioned Food Research Programme (see introduction), including food safety research to Irish food companies (in user-friendly form). It also helps to promote innovation. The dissemination procedures are listed in Fig. 2. These embrace (1) an inventory of the ongoing research projects in the Non-Commissioned Food Research Programme, (2) user-friendly technical updates on the results from the projects, (3) workshops on results from the projects, (4) selected technical publications and information bulletins, and lastly, (5) regular company visits by the three full time disseminators employed in the IRL-FLOW project. The major differences in the dissemination procedures of the FLAIR-FLOW and IRL-FLOW projects are the internet (FLAIR-FLOW only) and the company visits (IRL-FLOW only). Company visits are of crucial importance as they permit active dialogue, feedback, and the linking to the researchers doing the research (via the disseminator) all at the same time.

The three IRL-FLOW disseminators are strategically located at The National Food Centre (Dublin), The Dairy Products Research Centre (Fermoy) and at University College Cork, and each operates in a different region of the country.

IRL-FLOW Output

In the first year of IRL-FLOW an inventory containing all the projects in the Non-Commissioned Food Research Programme (NCFRP) was issued to 500

Irish companies and about 60 of the companies have been visited by the disseminators. The 'first round' of 81 technical one-page reports on the projects have been circulated and updates will be issued on an ongoing basis as results come on-stream. Nine workshops were held for the food industry on results from the NCFRP projects. Representatives from 140 food companies attended and overviews on two of the workshops have been published (Brennan 1997a,b).

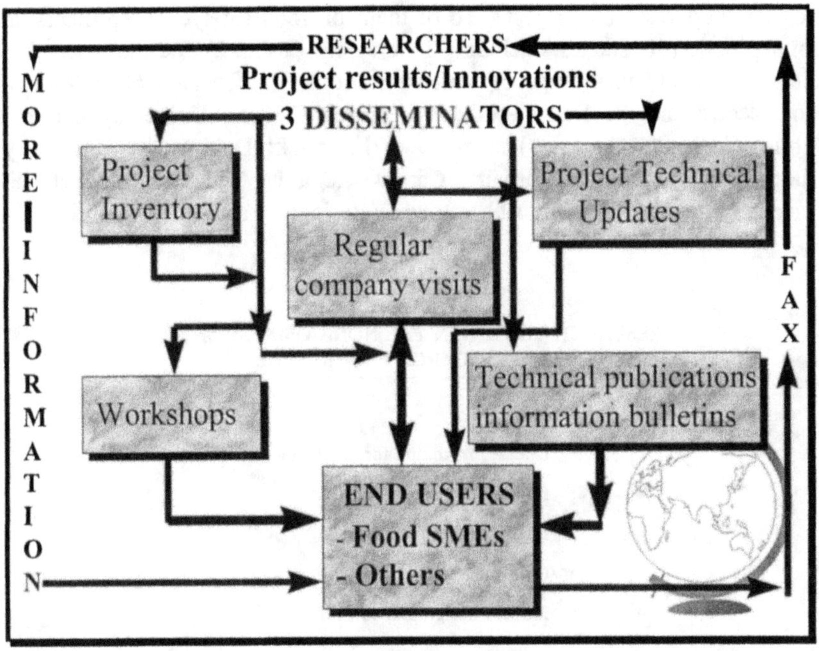

FIG. 2. *IRL-FLOW*: ROUTES FOR INFORMATION TRANSFER

An industry focused questionnaire was issued to all Irish food companies together with the project inventory. A 30% response rate has been achieved to date. The questionnaire addressed technical issues such as: in-company R & D, technology/information sources, the importance of product/process development, reasons why companies do not carry out R & D, level of interest in the 81 projects included in the project inventory, time scale of company R & D projects, R & D projects requiring further research, and the identification of key personnel interested in obtaining research results.

The data obtained from the food industry questionnaires have been entered into a tailor-made company database. As well as logging the above technical information, this database is updated on an ongoing basis with details gathered from company visits and other contacts. This includes the level of company interest in a particular project (which is graded), with emphasis on follow-up (in-depth) information. Early indications show that the database is producing some useful trends.

Non-Commissioned Food Research Programme

The Non-Commissioned Food Research Programme (NCFRP) embraces circa 85 food research projects, 16 of them on food safety. The projects are grouped under 10 themes, including food safety (Table 2) and the research is being carried out in a range of Irish institutions, i.e. Teagasc (The National Food Centre and the Dairy Products Research Centre); University Colleges Dublin, Cork and Galway; University of Limerick; Dublin City University; Trinity College Dublin; Forbairt; Carlow Regional Technical College; St. Vincent's Hospital, Dublin; Abbotstown Veterinary Laboratory, Dublin.

TABLE 2.
RESEARCH THEMES IN THE NON-COMMISSIONED FOOD RESEARCH PROGRAMME

- Food safety
- Cheese, fresh and fermented dairy products
- Food ingredients
- Beef and other meats
- Consumer foods
- Process design and control
- Nutrition
- Competitiveness
- Food industry waste
- Beverages

The titles of the 16 food safety projects are listed in Table 3. Technical updates are being issued on most of them with the exception of those which are in a start-up mode. The portfolio of food safety research projects is an indication of the high priority being given to safety in Ireland which is only proper for a 'good food island' serving the domestic and export markets.

TABLE 3.
FOOD SAFETY PROJECTS IN THE NON-COMMISSIONED FOOD RESEARCH PROGRAMME

- Chemical residues and pathogens
- Food safety - chemical residues and pathogens, and control strategies
- Control of enzymatic browning without the use of sulphites
- Microbiological safety of fresh ready-to-use vegetables
- Rapid detection of biogenic amines in food
- National food consumption survey for food chemical and nutrient intake
- Hen egg yoke: A source of novel antibacterial factors
- Detection of food spoilage/mycotoxigenic fungi and yeasts in food
- Development of residue analysis methods for veterinary drugs
- Food residue database - phase II
- Assessment and control of foodborne pathogens
- Pathogenic food poisoning bacteria as endophytic contaminants of food plants: a risk assessment
- Routine diagnostic tests for food pathogens
- Survival and virulence of *E. coli 0157* and *L. monocytogenes* in high risk foods
- Development of rapid detection methods for bacteria for use in HACCP programmes in the poultry meat industry
- The influence of hide cleaning, hide removal and evisceration on the spread of *E. coli 0157 H7* on beef carcasses

Information on IRL-FLOW

Contact any one of the three disseminators:

- Kevin Brennan, Teagasc, The National Food Centre, Dunsinea, Castleknock, Dublin 15, Ireland. Tel: + 353-1-8059564; Fax: + 353-1-8059550
- Gerard Dore, Teagasc, Dairy Products Research Centre, Fermoy, Co. Cork, Ireland. Tel: + 353-25-42282; Fax: + 353-25-42340
- Maria Creed, Faculty of Food Science and Technology, University College, Cork, Ireland. Tel: + 353-21-903138; Fax: + 353-21-276318

HIGHLIGHTING FOOD SAFETY RESEARCH

The FLAIR-FLOW and IRL-FLOW dissemination projects are highlighting the results from food safety research projects (both European and Irish) for the food industry and other end-users, including regulatory agencies/organisations. The dissemination is taking place as the projects are ongoing thereby ensuring a rapid and a 'latest state of the art' diffusion. This is of major importance as the rapid implementation of the results is essential in the area of food safety where consumer health and well-being may be at stake.

ACKNOWLEDGMENTS

We thank the European Union and the Irish Department of Agriculture and Food.

REFERENCES

ANON. 1994. FLAIR-FLOW: A model dissemination network. *Innovation and Technology Transfer*, *4*, 10–15.

BRENNAN, K. 1997a. Overview of food safety workshop at The National Food Centre. *Farm and Food* *7*(2), 35–36.

BRENNAN, K. 1997b. Recent developments in improving meat quality (Workshop overview). *Farm and Food* *7*(3), 10–12.

GORMLEY, T.R. 1992. FLAIR-FLOW EUROPE: a dissemination route to the food industry and consumers. *Trends in Food Science and Technology* *3*(5), 103–106.

GORMLEY, T.R. 1993. FLAIR-FLOW: a new and successful European approach to dissemination. *FLAIR-FLOW EUROPE Technical Circular* 113/93, 6 pages.

GORMLEY, T.R. 1994. FLAIR-FLOW: an overview of dissemination research in Europe. In: *Minimal Processing of Foods and Process Optimization - an Interface* (R.P. Singh and F.A.R. Oliveira, eds.), CRC Press, 505–516.

GORMLEY, T.R. 1995. RTD needs and opinions of European food SMEs. *Farm and Food* *5*(2), 27–30.

GORMLEY, T.R. 1996a. FLAIR-FLOW EUROPE: a novel dissemination project. *Food Technology International: Europe*, 14–18.

GORMLEY, T.R. 1996b. FLAIR-FLOW EUROPE: Disseminating food research results to European food SMEs. *FLAIR-FLOW EUROPE Technical Circular* 235/96, 6 pages.

GORMLEY, T.R. 1997. FLAIR-FLOW III: Providing key information for European Food SMEs. *FLAIR-FLOW EUROPE Technical Circular* 273/97, 2 pages.

CHAPTER 6

RESIDUES — A FOOD SAFETY PROBLEM?

MICHAEL O'KEEFFE and ORLA KENNEDY

Food Safety Department
Teagasc, The National Food Centre
Dunsinea, Castleknock, Dublin 15, Ireland

ABSTRACT

Considerable time, regulation and consumer concern is associated with the question of chemical residues in food. Potential residues in food span a broad range from natural contaminants (mycotoxins) through environmental contaminants (dioxins, PCBs), agrochemicals (nitrates, pesticides), veterinary drugs (anthelmintics, antibiotics), prohibited substances (hormonal growth promoters), chemicals arising in processing (nitrosamines), packaging components (plasticisers) to contaminants arising in domestic food preparation (heavy metals). The occurrence or avoidance of these chemicals as residues in food is to a greater or lesser extent under the control of the food producer, processor and consumer in the activities of growing/producing, treating, storing, processing, packaging and cooking. The fundamental question is to what extent do or can residues in food constitute a food safety hazard for the consumer. Many of these substances are regulated as to their use and as to their acceptable levels in food while others, by their nature, arise as more random occurrences and, as such, are less prone to regulation. Of particular concern to the producer, processor and retailer of food is what steps may be taken to ensure that the food supply is safe. Best practice in plant and animal husbandry by the producer, in sourcing of material and in control of food manufacturing by the processor, and in sourcing of food products by the retailer combine to assure the safety of food to the consumer. This paper describes the various classes of chemicals which can arise as residues in food, particularly agrochemicals and veterinary drugs, the usage patterns which decrease/increase the likelihood of the occurrence of residues at unacceptable levels, how and in what form(s) residues can occur in foods, and the contribution of food processing to a reduction or otherwise of residue levels in food consumed. Consideration will be given, also, to quantifying the risk posed by chemical residues in food and to a study of the results from a Residue Database and from residue monitoring/surveillance as an indicator of risk to the consumer.

INTRODUCTION

A very real contradiction exists in the developed world in the late 1990's regarding the risk to human health posed by residues of chemical contaminants in food. On the one hand the development of a range of agrochemicals and veterinary drugs, the intensification of agricultural production and the increase in industrialisation and associated environmental contamination points towards an increased exposure of the consumer to chemical residues from food and other sources. On the other hand, the regulation and control on use of agrochemicals and veterinary drugs, including the ongoing evaluation of their toxicity with ever better technologies, the extensive monitoring of the residue status of foods and the parallel controls on environmental pollution suggest that the status of the food supply should be much better than previously.

Yet the consumer looks increasingly for "pure" food, even for food produced according to the systems of yesteryear, and food producers, processors and retailers in their advertising and in their systems strive to deliver such "pure" food to the customer. In respect of residues in food, the emphasis is increasingly towards natural or "organic" systems for food production but, paradoxically, even if this goes some way to satisfy the concerns on agrochemical, veterinary drug and, possibly, industrial contaminants, it may not address the complete range of chemical contaminants, such as mycotoxins and natural toxins. The challenge, therefore, is to investigate with the currently-available knowledge whether the bulk of food available in the developed world and produced according to the conventional agricultural systems of the late 20th Century is likely to contain chemical residues posing a food safety risk for the consumer.

The scope of potential chemical residues in food is very great, ranging from natural contaminants, such as mycotoxins, through agrochemicals, veterinary drugs and prohibited growth promoting substances, to contaminants arising in processing, packaging, cooking and from the environment. Of major concern in this discussion are the chemicals arising in food as natural contaminants or from agricultural production. This paper will describe the different substances, their usage, potential occurrence in foods, their relative contribution to food toxicity, their fate in food processing/cooking and the profile of their actual occurrence in food, based on the results of residue surveys. The results from studies which are part of a Database on the Residue Status of Irish Foods (Kennedy and O'Keeffe 1996), together with the results from statutory monitoring programmes, will be used to indicate the actual residue content in Irish food products.

RESIDUES AND TOXICITY

Two sets of values are normally applied to the interpretation of residues in food; Maximum Residue Limits (MRLs) and Acceptable Daily Intake (ADI) values. The MRL is the maximum concentration of a residue, expressed as mg per kg food, legally permitted in or on food commodities and animal feeds. MRL values for a residue are particular to each food or food type. The Acceptable Daily Intake (ADI) value is an estimate of the amount of residue, expressed as mg per kg bodyweight, that can be ingested daily over a lifetime without appreciable health risk. The ADI is based on a toxicological evaluation, under a range of criteria, of the chemical and is based on the no-adverse-effect level in test animals and contains safety factors to account for inter-species differences (normally × 10) and differences between humans (normally × 10), such as vulnerable (sick) individuals, infants, elderly, etc.

Typically, MRLs are not set at levels at which ingestion of an appropriate quantity of the particular food, containing residue at the MRL, would result in the ADI value being exceeded. For some residues and some foods, the MRL values are such that even in situations where they would be substantially exceeded there is no risk of the ADI being exceeded. On the other hand, for certain residue and food combinations, the ADI would be exceeded where the residue level in the food is slightly above the MRL. The relationship between the MRL for a particular food/residue combination and the ADI for the residue is somewhat complex. An estimate of intake of the particular food is used to determine whether food containing residue at a level above the MRL is likely to result in the ADI being exceeded; such estimates are based on average intake. Except in extreme cases, where residues in food are at acute toxicity levels, occasional ingestion of food with residue in excess of the MRL, or even occasional exceeding of the ADI for a residue, are unlikely to cause any adverse effect when one considers both the high safety factors applied to ADI values and the fact that they are based on a lifetime ingestion of the residue.

Incidences of observable toxic effects due to chemical residues in food are largely localized and occur over relatively short time periods. In most cases they are due to environmental contamination of food (such as the contamination of fish with mercury giving rise to Minamata disease in Japan), the misuse of particular agrochemicals or veterinary drugs (such as the acute toxicity effects observed on ingestion of cucumber treated with Aldicarb in Ireland in 1992), and the use of prohibited substances where no recommended treatment regime is available (such as the incidences of toxic reactions due to clenbuterol residues in liver in Spain and in France during 1990). For all of these, and similar food toxicity incidents, there was the capacity to respond to the observed clinical symptoms and identify the causative agent specifically in the food. Subsequent removal of the contaminated food resulted in the incidences of toxicity being removed, also.

More difficult to associate definitely with a particular chemical residue in food are clinical observations over an extended period of time. A good example of such a situation was the reported precocious sexual development observed in young children in Puerto Rico in the period 1978/1981 (Comas 1982; De Rodriguez and Toro-Sola 1982). The details of this incident were that the symptoms were observed in over 600 children under eight years of age over a 10-year period. The original authors of these clinical reports suspected food additives or contaminants to be responsible, in the form of oestrogenic substances, and the blame was laid at the door of anabolic agents such as diethylstilboestrol and zeranol which were widely available and used in meat production. However, it was pointed out that other oestrogenic agents might be responsible, such as the mycotoxin zearalenone, and that, since all oestrogenic substances act in a similar fashion (through receptor binding in target organs), the observed clinical effects might be due to a combination of oestrogenic substances in food (Schoental 1983).

Even more difficult still to assign as contributing to human ill-health are nonclinical chronic effects due to low levels of residues in foods. The concern that such residues may contribute in an accumulative way to human ill-health is quite prevalent. Whether there is any basis for such a concern is largely unprovable but it warrants and underlines the necessity to keep chemical residues in food to the lowest level possible. It is about how to achieve the lowest level possible that most of the debate hinges and where there is, at least apparently, a conflict between intensive agriculture to produce relatively cheap food for all the people and a good return to the producers versus extensive, "organic" systems of agriculture in which food safety and wholesomeness is claimed to be secure. As is the case with many things, the resolution is a compromise: reduced use of chemicals in agriculture and systems to prevent the occurrence of residues in food at levels of concern to the population.

MYCOTOXINS

Mycotoxins are considered to be some of the most toxic chemicals occurring as natural contaminants of animal feed and human food. They are produced by moulds growing on plant products such as grains, nuts and fruit. Human exposure to mycotoxins may arise, therefore, either directly from plant products or indirectly through meat and milk from animals given feed containing high levels of mycotoxins. Some of the most important mycotoxins are the aflatoxins B_1, B_2, G_1, G_2 (and the derivative aflatoxin M_1 in milk), ochratoxin A, sterigmatocystin, zearalenone, patulin and citrinin.

A recent survey of animal feed ingredients in the United Kingdom identified aflatoxin B_1 as the most common contaminant in rice bran, maize products, palm kernals and cottonseed, and ochratoxin A and citrinin as the most common contaminants in wheat and barley (Scudamore *et al.* 1997). Of particular interest as contaminants in foods of animal origin are aflatoxin M_1 in milk and dairy products and ochratoxin A in pork. Very stringent regulations have been introduced for aflatoxin M_1 in milk and dairy products with MRLs of 0.01 to 0.05 ppb in milk being set by a number of countries. Ochratoxin A has been implicated in causing kidney damage to pigs and ingestion of ochratoxin A, from cereals and pulses, has been found to cause a chronic, progressive disease (Balkan endemic nephropathy) in humans. Results of surveys carried out by The National Food Centre on the incidence of aflatoxin M_1 in dairy powders (Fig. 1) and of ochratoxin A in pig kidney (Fig. 2) show that, while the mycotoxins occur at low levels in many samples tested, these levels are well below MRLs (or other safe limits) and, as such, do not pose a health risk for consumers. For example, in the case of aflatoxin M_1 the safe limit for dairy powders (derived from the proposed EU MRL for milk of 0.05 ppb) would be of the order of 0.5 and 1.75 ppb for skim milk and casein powders, respectively. The results of such studies suggest that the major potential source of exposure of consumers to mycotoxins is from plant foods, rather than from foods of animal origin.

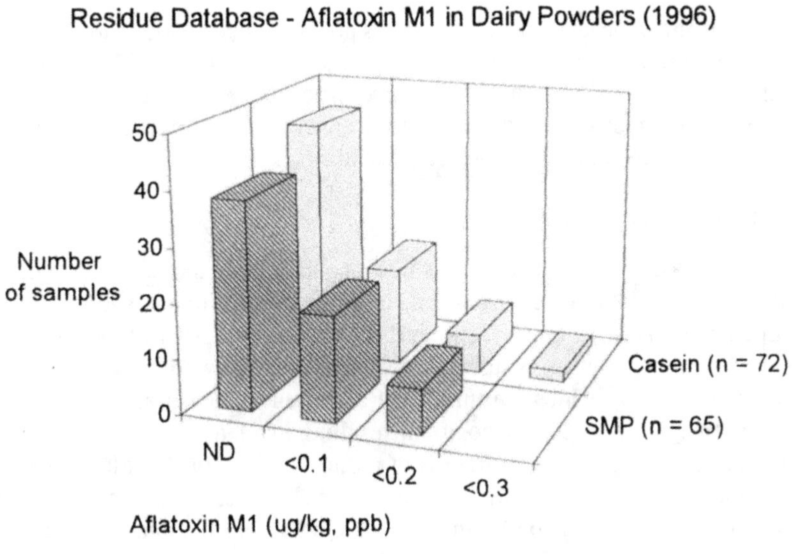

FIG. 1. AFLATOXIN M1 IN DAIRY POWDER SAMPLES OBTAINED FROM THE IRISH DAIRY INDUSTRY IN 1996 (RESIDUE DATABASE STUDY)

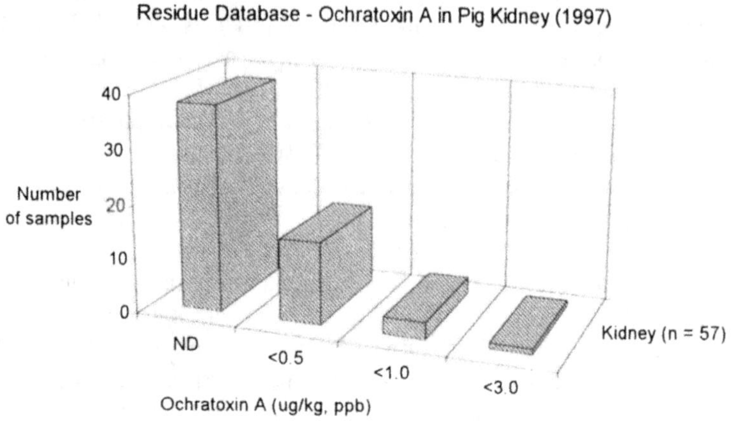

FIG. 2. OCHRATOXIN A IN PIG KIDNEY SAMPLES OBTAINED FROM THE IRISH PORK INDUSTRY IN 1997 (RESIDUE DATABASE STUDY)

AGROCHEMICALS

The main agrochemicals of concern as potential food residues are fertilizers and pesticides. The use of fertilizers and pesticides has increased throughout the latter half of the 20th century with intensification of agriculture and food production. Currently, considerable efforts are being made to limit and decrease the use of agrochemicals, particularly fertilizers.

Fertilizers

In the case of fertilizers there is much concern over the increase in nitrate (and nitrite) levels in the environment, in grass, in plant foods, and in foods of animal origin, such as milk. High levels of nitrate-nitrogen in food and water are undesirable because, while nitrate itself is of low toxicity, it may be converted to nitrite which, in turn, may act as an oxidising agent converting blood haemoglobin to methaemoglobin resulting in a reduced oxygen supply to body tissues. This effect of nitrate is of particular concern for infants who are biochemically disposed towards both an enhanced conversion of nitrate to nitrite and a reduced reconversion of methaemoglobin to haemoglobin. In addition, nitrite can react with constituents of the food to form N-nitroso compounds which have been identified as potential carcinogens. Nitrate and nitrite are used for meat curing and N-nitroso compounds have been found to occur in many varieties of meat preserved using nitrite (Walters 1992). The combination of nitrate and nitrite occurring in food both from agricultural use of nitrogen-containing fertilizers and from food additive use indicates that a reduction in the overall intake of nitrate/nitrite is desirable.

The dietary intake of nitrate has been calculated for the United Kingdom (Meah *et al.* 1994) and The Netherlands (Brussaard *et al.* 1996) on the basis of Total Diet Study data. In both countries, the main contributors to nitrate in the diet were identified as vegetables. In the case of nitrite, which was calculated also for the United Kingdom, vegetables were also the major contributor to dietary intake, even though some cured meats contained higher concentrations of nitrite. The estimated total dietary intake of nitrate in the United Kingdom was 54 mg/person/day and for nitrite was 4.2 mg/person/day (Table 1). These figures were considered to be well within the EC Scientific Committee for Food (SCF) ADI for nitrate (0-219 mg/60 kg person/day), but to be just within the SCF temporary ADI for nitrite (0-4.2 mg/60 kg person/day) (Commission of the European Communities Scientific Committee for Food 1992). In the case of the Dutch study, which was confined to nitrate, it was found that while mean intake of nitrate never exceeded the ADI, individual intakes were found to be above the ADI in 3-23% of subjects and this was higher in the younger age groups. The data from the Total Diet Study in the United Kingdom and The Netherlands for nitrate/nitrite suggest that, while intake of these chemicals on a mean population basis may be within the acceptable daily intake, there may be a section of the population, defined in terms of age or dietary habits, who are potentially consuming nitrate/nitrite above the acceptable level.

TABLE 1.
NITRATE AND NITRITE IN FOOD - TOTAL DIET STUDY (UK)

	Content (mg/kg)		Dietary intake (mg/person/day)			Acceptable Daily Intake (mg/person/day)
	vegetables	meats	vegetables	other foods	total	
Nitrate	10 - 3000	<0.8 - 410	41	13	54	0 - 219
Nitrite	<3 - 60	<0.5 - 130	2.1	2.1	4.2	0 - 4.2

(adapted from Meah *et al.* 1994)

In milk, nitrate levels of 0.3-12 mg/kg can be expected and in dried milk products 10-30 mg/kg can be observed, according to a recent IDF report (Bluthgen *et al.* 1997). A study at The National Food Centre on nitrate/nitrite levels in skim milk and casein powders showed that, while most samples contained nitrate at below 30 mg/kg, some samples contained nitrate in excess of this level (Fig. 3). In the case of nitrite, levels were generally at less than 3 mg/kg but some samples of casein powders contained levels at 3-6 mg/kg. It has been suggested that the temperatures of combustion of natural gases, used in the manufacturing/drying of these products, may be sufficiently high for the combination of nitrogen and oxygen to produce nitrate and nitrite (Walters 1991).

Pesticides

Pesticides have been applied to crops and to animals for many years to control pests, fungi and weeds. They are an integral part of high-yield, intensive agriculture. Pesticides are used at all stages of agriculture and food production beginning with pretreatment of fields (weed control) and housing (pest control), through crop (pest, weed and fungus control) and animal (pest control) treatments, to treatment of harvested food (pest and fungus control). In addition, pesticides used in crop production may contribute to subsequent animal exposure due to use of the crop as a feedstuff.

There are hundreds of pesticides of different chemistry, many of them grouped into classes of similar chemical structure and/or mode of action. Examples include organochlorine, organophosphorous and carbamate pesticides. The most desirable pesticide is one which has high efficacy (i.e. low dose requirement), highly specific toxicity (i.e. eliminates pest only) and very low persistence beyond its effective period. Developments in pesticides have been away from more persistent types such as organochlorine pesticides to the less persistent organophosphorous pesticides. Indeed, the use of organochlorine pesticides as active ingredients in plant protection products has been prohibited by the European Commission and the number of incidents and levels of such pesticides found as residues in foods from within the EU has decreased. Where residues of organochlorine pesticides are found in food products, these are due, generally, to persistent residues in soil or storage containers/buildings, to food/feed products from countries where organochlorine pesticides are still used in agriculture, to pesticide preparations containing organochlorines as impurities, or possibly to illegal use (Pesticide Control Service 1997).

All pesticides allowed for use in agriculture must be authorized for use in Ireland by the Pesticide Control Service of the Department of Agriculture and Food under EU regulations. These regulations require that pesticides authorized for use in food production have associated with them ADI and MRL values and that their use, in terms of rate of application to particular crops/animals and withdrawal periods, is specified. Where the use of a pesticide product is according to the authorisation, i.e. according to good agricultural practice, residues in the resulting food should not occur above the specified MRL for that food. Good agricultural practice (GAP) is the use as authorized for the pesticide under practical conditions necessary for effective control of the target pests.

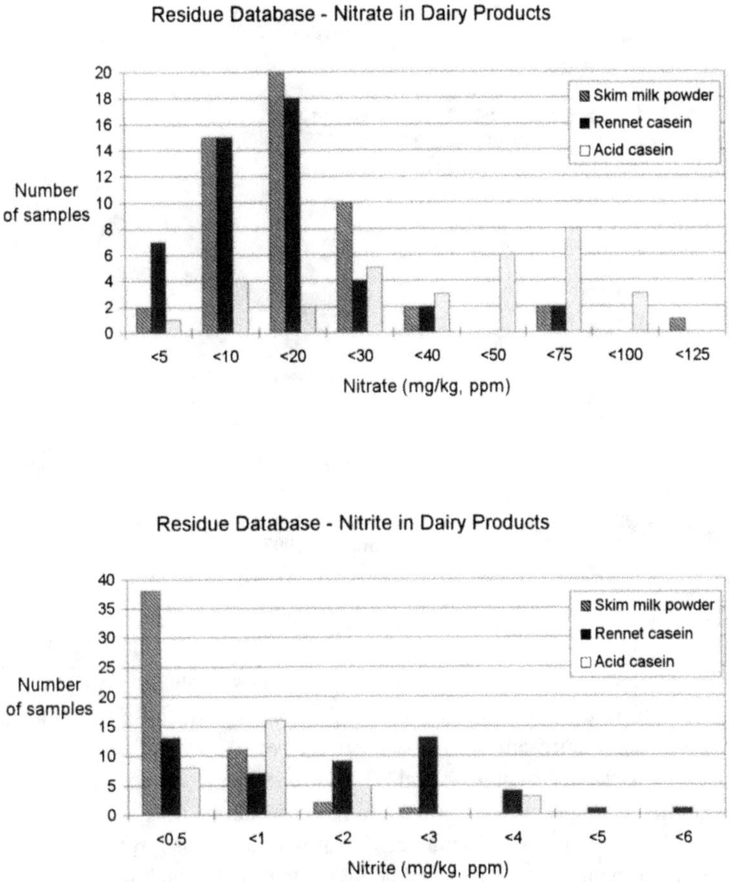

FIG. 3. NITRATE AND NITRITE CONTENT OF DAIRY POWDERS OBTAINED FROM THE IRISH DAIRY INDUSTRY IN 1997 (RESIDUE DATABASE STUDY)
(Skim milk powder, n = 52; Rennet casein, n = 48; Acid casein, n = 32)

Results for the pesticide residue-monitoring programme in Ireland (and other European countries) in recent years demonstrate the actual health risk to consumers from pesticide residues in food. The Pesticide Control Service of the Department of Agriculture and Food report that while the overall incidence of residue-positive samples is at approximately 40-50% of samples of fruit and vegetables, cereals and meat and dairy products tested during the years 1994 to 1996, the residue levels are generally below the MRLs. Only 31 samples, or 1.9%, of the total of 1667 fruit, vegetable and cereal samples tested over this 3-year period contained residues above the MRLs (Fig. 4). In meat and dairy products no residue levels in excess of the MRLs were determined, from a sampling of 1527 samples over the 3-year period (Pesticide Control Service 1997).

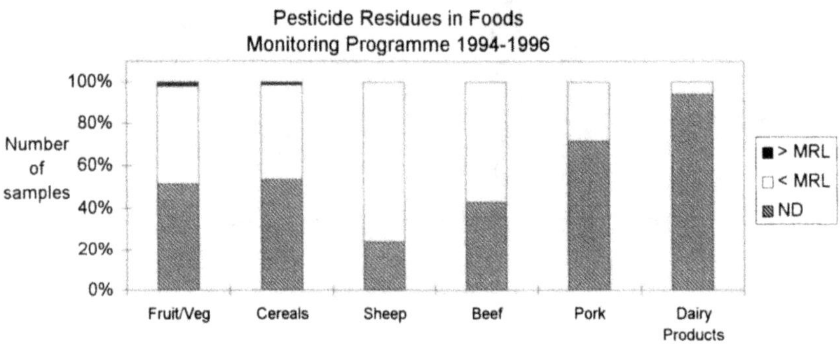

FIG. 4. PESTICIDE RESIDUES IN FOODS - RESULTS FOR MONITORING PROGRAM IN IRELAND, 1994 - 1996
(Adapted from Pesticide Control Service, Department of Agriculture, Food and Forestry, 1997)

Where the residue levels determined in the 31 samples of fruit, vegetables and cereals are interpreted in terms of the ADI values for these pesticides, only in 4 incidences (representing an occurrence of 0.24% of the total 3-year sampling) were the ADI values equalled or exceeded. Considering the issues of safety factors, average intake figures and noncontinuous intake of the particular residue-positive food, these incidences do not indicate any real risk to human health. Indeed, apart from direct and acute toxic effects, such as may arise from abuse/misuse of pesticides in crops, there is no indication of a general risk to human health from pesticide residues. One of the problems with an abuse/misuse situation, such as the incident in which Aldicarb was applied to cucumbers, is that the normal monitoring programme is unlikely to find the problem. In that case, the first sign of a problem was the acute toxic effect observed in consumers; however, the value and importance of the monitoring programme is that it can give early warning of potential problems with a particular pesticide/food combination, indicate some recurring problems with imported foods and, most importantly, give reassurance to the consumer that pesticide residues in foods are at levels unlikely to cause adverse health effects.

VETERINARY DRUGS

Veterinary drugs, similarly to pesticides, are regulated in a positive manner by authorisation to market a product from the Irish Medicines Board, operating according to the European Commission directives on veterinary medicinal products (Council of the European Communities 1981a,b), and with MRL and ADI values established. Apart from the authorisation to market particular veterinary drugs, such as antibiotics and anthelmintics, European Commission and Irish regulations ban the use of certain substances, particularly growth-promoting substances such as anabolic hormones and repartitioning agents (S.I. No. 218 of 1988, S.I. No. 171 of 1990).

Veterinary drugs are allowed for use within the EU only where a MRL has been established. The main veterinary drugs of interest are the prohibited growth-promoting agents, antibiotics used for prophylactic and therapeutic purposes and antiparasiticides. Within Ireland, in extensive production systems such as beef and sheep meat, potential use of drugs would be largely from growth-promoting agents and antiparasiticides; antibiotics are likely to be used only on individual (sick) animals not going for slaughter. In intensive production systems such as pig and poultry meat, potential use of drugs would be largely from antibiotics, since these may be used widely to prevent (prophylactic) or treat (therapeutic) disease in herds and flocks. In the case of milk and dairy products, the main source of potential residues would be from antibiotics used in mastitis treatment.

Growth-Promoting Substances

Within the class of growth-promoting substances there are a range of chemicals which might be used illegally: steroids, both "natural" and "synthetic" and related chemicals such as zeranol and stilbenes which have an anabolic, or growth-promoting, effect through their androgenic or oestrogenic effects, thyreostatic hormones which influence growth through their effect on the metabolic activity of the animal and β-agonists or repartitioning agents which influence growth through directing the energy from feed into muscle tissue growth rather than fat tissue growth — i.e. enhanced efficiency of lean meat production. Within the EU, all of these substances are prohibited for use to influence growth of animals.

All EU countries have extensive monitoring programmes in place to check on the use of these substances in meat (largely beef and veal) production and on the presence of residues of these substances in edible tissues. The β-agonists (clenbuterol) are a particular problem in that the effective dose for growth promotion is some multiples of the therapeutic dose (i.e. where this veterinary drug is used legitimately for treatment of bronchopulmonary conditions). Because the redistribution effect is reversed when the drug is withdrawn, the illegal use of β-agonists (generally in feed) to obtain the growth promotion effect requires that they be used up to a short period before slaughter. Residues may occur, therefore, in edible tissues at levels capable of inducing toxic effects, as for example, in the incidents reported from Spain and France (Martinez-Navarro 1990; Pulce *et al.* 1991); however, because of the extensive monitoring and control measures in the EU the occurrence of toxic residue levels in meat has not been widely observed.

In the case of anabolic agents there is an interesting divergence of view on their use between the EU and most other countries (e.g. U.S., Australia, New Zealand, Argentina). Whereas in the EU the use of all anabolic agents is prohibited, in other countries certain of these drugs such as the natural hormones (oestradiol, progesterone and testosterone) and the synthetic anabolic agents, trenbolone and zeranol, are permitted. Other anabolic agents, such as the stilbenes, are prohibited in many countries because of toxicity evaluation which demonstrated that they have carcinogenic potency. Anabolic agents, such as nortestosterone, methyltestosterone and ethinyloestradiol, are generally prohibited for use as growth promoters. In the case of the natural hormones and the synthetic anabolic agents, trenbolone and zeranol, a very thorough evaluation of their toxicity by the FAO/WHO JECFA committee demonstrated that, when used according to good agricultural/veterinary practice, the residue levels resulting in edible tissues posed no appreciable risk to human health (WHO 1988). Since these products are not orally active, the approved dosage route is via slow-release implants deposited in nonedible tissue such as the ear, from which site they can produce a growth promotion effect for 3 to 12 months.

The different views on these anabolic agents has led to serious difficulties in international trade between the EU and other countries and these problems are by no means fully resolved. Reports in Italy (Loizzo *et al.* 1984) and Puerto Rico (Comas 1982; De Rodriguez and Toro-Sola 1982; Schoental 1983) in the early 1980s suggested a linkage of hormonally-related developments in prepubertal children to oestrogenic substances in the diet, possibly mycotoxins and/or anabolic agents. Otherwise, there have been few if any reports of toxic effects on humans which might be related to residues of anabolic agents in meat; however, particularly because of the black-market situation within the EU, there is ongoing danger that growth-promoting substances, alone or as cocktails, may be used and may be applied to animals in sites which could give rise to residues in edible tissues. For this reason monitoring programmes to check on the occurrence of these chemicals as residues in edible tissues are important.

A survey of retail-purchased beef steak and liver from EU countries undertaken by the *Association des Consommateurs - Test Achats* in 1994 found a relatively high incidence of residue-positive samples for both anabolic agents and β-agonists (Remy and Debeuckelaere 1994). The incidence of positive samples varied from 0% for anabolic agents and β-agonists in Denmark to 6.7% for anabolic agents in Belgium and 23 and 36% for β-agonists (clenbuterol) in Belgium and Spain, respectively (Fig. 5). The situation in Ireland was intermediate with 2.7% of samples found positive for anabolic agents and 1.7% for clenbuterol. Recent results for Ireland's national monitoring programme for the period January to September 1997 indicate a confirmed residue-positive incidence of 0.2% for anabolic agents and 0% for clenbuterol (Table 2).

In assessing the risk to human health from residues of growth-promoting substances it is important to consider that the lowest level of residue occurs, generally, in muscle tissue (with the liver, typically, being the edible tissue with the highest concentration). For anabolic agents, objective toxicological evaluation has found that some of these do not give rise to residues of concern in edible tissue when used correctly. In the case of β-agonists the levels of clenbuterol found in bovine liver (Spain) were at up to 300 ppb and in veal liver (France) were at up to 500 ppb. These levels are indicative of a high over-dosage to achieve the illicit growth-enhancing effect.

Given that suitable monitoring and control systems are in place, together with adequate penalties to deal with cases of abuse, the likelihood of growth-promoting substances arising in edible tissues at residue levels likely to cause serious toxic effects to humans must be considered to be low. This view is supported by the absence of any reported incidences of toxic effects on consumers in Ireland which could be linked to ingestion of edible tissues containing such residues; however, the incidences in Spain and France related to β-agonists and the incidences in Italy and Puerto Rico possibly related to anabolic agents confirm the necessity for constant control and monitoring of the meat supply to prevent such occurrences.

Antibiotics

A wide range of antibacterials and antibiotics are available for use in animal husbandry. Some of the more important classes of these drugs are sulphonamides, β-lactams (e.g. penicillin), tetracyclines, aminoglycosides (e.g. streptomycin), macrolides (e.g. erythromycin), peptide antibiotics (e.g. virginiamycin) and ionophores (e.g. monensin). The latter two classes of drugs are used primarily as feed additive growth promoters rather than as therapeutic antibiotics and their use, in terms of dosage and period of use, is regulated by specific European Commission and national regulations. Certain antibiotics previously used in animal husbandry are now prohibited for use in food-producing animals; chloramphenicol, because of its potential toxicity for susceptible humans, and the nitrofurans, because of their mutagenic, carcinogenic and bound-residue characteristics.

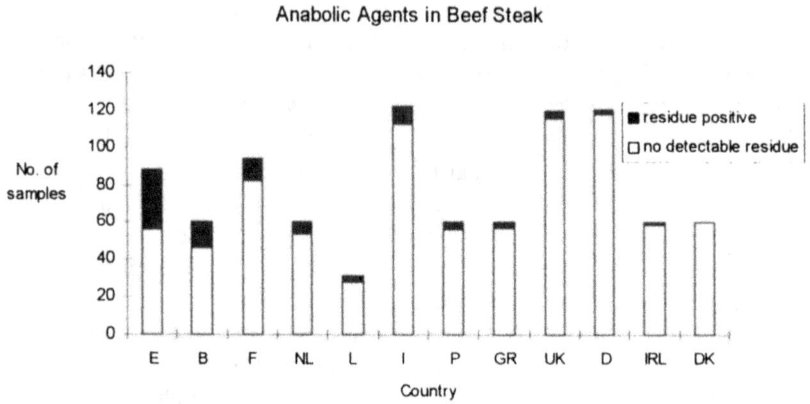

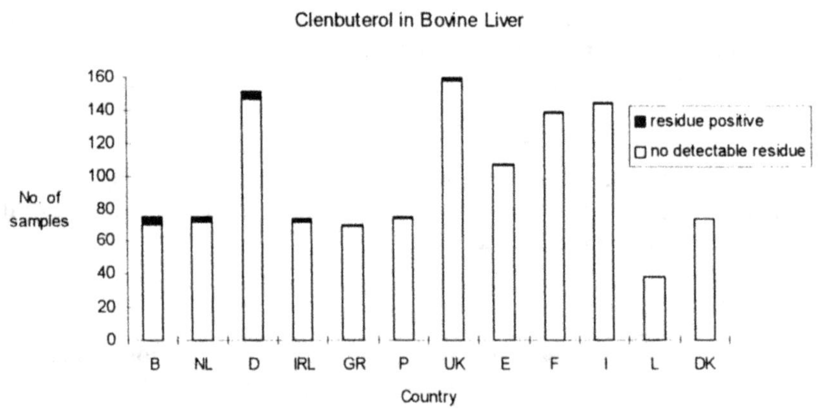

FIG. 5. RESIDUES OF GROWTH-PROMOTING SUBSTANCES IN MEAT — RESULTS OF RETAIL STUDY BY CONSUMERS ASSOCIATION 1994
(adapted from Remy and Debeuckelaere 1994)

TABLE 2.
RESULTS OF MONITORING PROGRAMME FOR RESIDUES OF VETERINARY DRUGS IN MEAT, JANUARY - SEPTEMBER 1997

	Number of samples tested (positive)			
Substance	Bovine	Ovine	Porcine	Poultry
Hormones	12,890 (24)	113 (0)	148 (0)	nt
Clenbuterol	51,020 (0)	55 (0)	50 (0)	nt
Antibiotics	3,939 (45)	331 (2)	39,232 (651)	142 (0)

(adapted from Department of Agriculture and Food 1997), nt - not tested

Antibiotic residues can occur in edible tissues and in milk primarily from situations where insufficient withdrawal periods are observed between treatment and slaughter or use of milk. Similarly to other chemicals, maximum residue limits are established for antibiotics and withdrawal periods are specified for each approved use and animal species such that the MRL will not be exceeded. A survey of retail-purchased pork and poultry meat from EU countries undertaken by the *Association des Consommateurs - Test Achats* in 1996 (Debeuckelaere and Remy 1996) found a high incidence of residue-positive meat from some countries, including Ireland (Fig. 6). The survey found 17% of Irish pork samples to be residue-positive for tetracycline antibiotics using screening tests such as the official EU Four Plate test and immunoassays. Analyses of Irish pork for tetracycline antibiotic residues undertaken during 1996, as part of the Residue Database project, confirmed the presence of chlortetracycline residues in muscle and kidney samples (Table 3). Residues at levels exceeding the MRL were found in 5% of meat samples tested, using specific high performance liquid chromatography (HPLC) analysis.

A particular problem with use of screening tests for residue determination is that the residue tests may be over-sensitive for the MRL values for certain antibiotic residues. In such a case, samples will be determined as positive where they contain residues at lower than the MRL. This is a real consumer problem in that, notwithstanding a toxicity evaluation which specifies an ADI value and

MRLs for particular foods which respect this ADI in terms of the contribution of the foods to the diet, sensitive methods may identify samples as residue-positive where the residue content is considerably below the MRL. Residue-positive samples are not attractive to consumers even where the residue concentration is objectively declared to be safe.

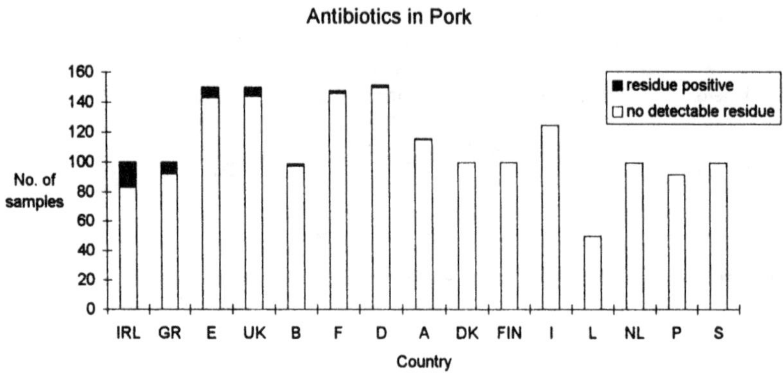

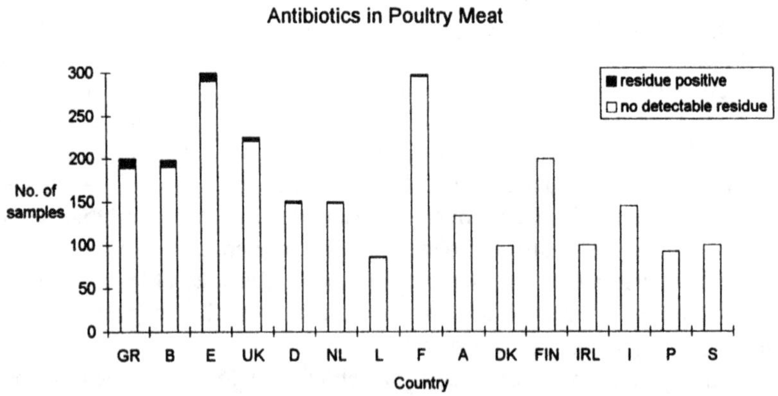

FIG. 6. RESIDUES OF ANTIBIOTICS IN MEAT – RESULTS OF RETAIL STUDY BY CONSUMERS ASSOCIATION 1996
(adapted from Debeuckelaere and Remy, 1996)

TABLE 3.
CHLORTETRACYCLINE ANTIBIOTICS IN TISSUE SAMPLES OBTAINED FROM THE IRISH PORK INDUSTRY IN 1996 (RESIDUE DATABASE STUDY)

	Number (%) of samples at each residue level		
Sample (number)	ND	<MRL	>MRL
Meat (140)	98 (70%)	35 (25%)	7 (5%)
Kidney (57)	16 (28%)	41 (72%)	0 (0%)

MRLs: 100 ppb (muscle), 600 ppb (kidney)

In the case of antibiotics, an additional problem stems from the hotly-debated question of bacterial resistance and to what extent the use of antibiotics in intensive animal production systems contributes to this problem. Because the same antibiotics, largely, are used in human medicine as are used in treatment of animals, it is not possible to easily establish the contribution from each source to the development of bacterial resistance. Concern has been expressed as to the possible exposure of consumers to resistant bacteria present in meat or other edible tissues (WHO 1997), but this is a microbiological hazard, primarily, rather than a chemical residue one. Residues of antibiotics, *per se*, present in edible tissues at levels below the MRLs are not considered a causative agent for induction of bacterial resistance; this is so because ADIs (which the MRLs respect) are increasingly set on the basis of establishing minimum inhibitory concentration (MIC) values. MIC values are the concentration of antibiotic which has no inhibitory effect on the bacteria in the human gut.

The significant reduction in the incidence of residue-positive pork during 1997 (Table 2), in response to intensive testing and controls at factory level and by the Department of Agriculture and Food, indicates that it is possible to produce "residue-free" (meaning residues absent or nondetectable) meat through application of good veterinary practice (GVP) in the use of antibiotics, such as application of adequate withdrawal periods; however, in the case of antibiotics (as with many other veterinary drugs) the constant improvement in residue-testing technologies, particularly in improved sensitivity, makes it more difficult for producers to demonstrate that their meat is "residue-free". In the case of pork production, it would appear that some countries, such as Denmark, Sweden and Finland, are able to produce largely "residue-free" meat and this should be possible also for the Irish industry, but it may only be achievable with some fairly fundamental changes in production practices towards enhanced disease status of pig herds, much more controlled use of antibiotics, use of alternative treatments such as immunisation and radical changes to the structure of pig production units and the movement of pigs through such units. In the 1980's, when the milk withholding times specified for a number of dairy cow antibiotic treatments for mastitis were found to be inadequate, resulting in residue-positive milk, new veterinary products were readily developed. These experiences indicate that the achievement of "residue-free" milk and meat are possible and must be the aim of producers so as to satisfy consumer demands.

Anthelmintics

Anthelmintics are veterinary drugs used for treatment of animals against parasites such as fluke, worms and warble-fly. These drugs, generally benzimidazoles, organophosphorous compounds and avermectins, are used in all species of animals but mostly in cattle and sheep. With proper usage, these drugs should not arise as residues in meat because treatment for parasites is unlikely to occur close to slaughter; however, incidences of residues in food have been observed, usually in situations of widespread use as, for example, organophosphorous compounds in milk at low levels during compulsory warble-fly treatment (O'Keeffe *et al.* 1983) or ivermectin in salmon arising from use of this chemical to deal with large-scale sea-lice infestations. A similar situation arises for anthelmintics as for antibiotics in terms of observance of withdrawal periods to ensure that residues in food are nondetectable or below the MRLs.

CONSUMER EXPOSURE TO RESIDUES

In evaluating the potential exposure of the consumer to chemical residues in food a number of factors come into play which may increase or decrease this potential exposure and the associated risk. We have discussed already the question of more vulnerable individuals, such as infants, the elderly, sick people and those with increased susceptibility to certain chemical residues. In addition, there are those individuals who do not consume the "average" diet (on which MRLs are based) and those in whose diet significant quantities of particular foods may be supplied from a particular source. The inter-individual safety factor (× 10) used in deriving an ADI value for a particular chemical is intended to allow for these differences.

On the positive side, there are factors which act to reduce the actual exposure of the consumer to some chemical residues. In the case of pesticides in plant foods (where most of the significant pesticide residue levels occur), commercial processing, domestic preparation, and cooking tend to reduce the levels of organochlorine, organophosphorous and carbamate pesticides ingested by the consumer (Zabik 1987). Since much of the residue contamination is found primarily on the surface, peeling and, to a lesser extent, washing were found to be effective. The effect of cooking (115.5C) resulted in losses of pesticides and such losses were greater, generally, for organophosphorous and carbamate than for organochlorine pesticides, although differences were observed, also, within each class of pesticides (Table 4).

TABLE 4.
SUMMARY OF EFFECT OF PROCESSING ON PESTICIDE LEVELS IN FOOD (FRUITS AND VEGETABLES)

Procedure	Reduction in pesticide content (%)		
	Organochlorine pesticides	Organophosphorous pesticides	Carbamate pesticides
Commercial preparation	50 - 100	39 - 100	58 - 100
Home preparation	14 - 100	11 - 100	11 - 92
Cooking (115.5 C)	7 - 33	17 - 100	45 - 100

(adapted from Zabik 1987)

In the case of mycotoxins, studies have been undertaken on the effect of cooking on aflatoxin B1 in herbs and spices (MacDonald and Castle 1996) and on ochratoxin A in a range of foods such as baked goods, coffee and meat products (Battaglia *et al.* 1996). A summary of the findings from these studies are that aflatoxin levels are not reduced by domestic cooking with either microwave or conventional gas oven heating and that the general picture for ochratoxin A is that it survives most food processing to quite an appreciable degree.

A series of interesting studies have been undertaken by researchers at the Food Science Laboratory, MAFF, Norwich, UK on the effects of cooking on a range of veterinary drug residues such as the β-agonist, clenbuterol (Rose *et al.* 1995a), the antibiotics, sulphamethazine (Rose *et al.* 1995c) and oxytetracycline (Rose *et al.* 1996) and the anthelmintics, levamisole (Rose *et al.* 1995b) and oxfendazole (Rose *et al.* 1997). In summary (Table 5), clenbuterol, sulphamethazine and levamisole were largely unaffected by any form of cooking leading the authors to conclude that data from measurements on raw tissue are suitable for use in consumer exposure estimates. In the case of oxytetracycline substantial net losses of 35-94 % were observed, while in the case of oxfendazole the situation was unclear largely due to the instability of the residue and its nonhomogeneous distribution in the tissue. A similar study on the nitrofuran antibacterial, furazolidone, found that the protein bound metabolite, 3-amino-2-oxazolidinone, was stable during cooking and residue levels were not significantly reduced (McCracken and Kennedy 1997).

TABLE 5.
SUMMARY OF EFFECT OF PROCESSING ON VETERINARY DRUG LEVELS IN FOOD (EDIBLE TISSUES)

	Net change (%) on cooking				
Veterinary Drug	Microwave	Frying	Roasting	Boiling	Grilling
Clenbuterol, liver	+2	+1	nt	nt	nt
Sulfamethazine, muscle	+2	-3	+8	-1	-30
Oxytetracycline, muscle	-80	-49	-94	-75	-39
Levamisole, muscle	-7	+13	nt	-6	-11

(adapted from Rose et al. 1995/96), nt - not tested

In summary, the effects of food processing, preparation and cooking may have an important effect in reducing the consumer exposure to residues of pesticides in fruit and vegetables, but in the case of mycotoxins and veterinary drugs, there is generally no appreciable reduction in the potential exposure of the consumer to these chemicals if they occur as residues in food.

CONCLUSIONS

Chemical residues in food are an issue of concern to the consumer and this concern is supported by the incidences of toxic effects which have been associated, directly or indirectly, with residues in food. Residue monitoring/surveillance programmes and research studies, such as the Residue Database project, provide important information on the actual position on residues in food. Apart from providing information on the residue status of the food supply, these studies can identify areas of concern leading to the adoption of practices to eliminate or reduce the level of residues in food. While there have been incidences of residues in food causing toxic effects to consumers, these have been relatively few, and the results of residue monitoring/surveillance indicate that, generally, chemical residues are not a significant food safety problem; however, residues may occur at levels which are considered to be undesirable, and/or which exceed permitted levels, and food production practices must aim to reduce or eliminate residues from food.

ACKNOWLEDGEMENTS

The research project, Database on the Residue Status of Irish Foods, was partly funded by grant aid under the Food Sub-programme for Industrial Development which is administered by the Department of Agriculture and Food, Republic of Ireland and supported by national and EU funds. The contribution of P. Byrne, F. Farrell and E. Horne to these studies is gratefully acknowledged.

REFERENCES

BATTAGLIA, R., HATZOLD, T. and KROES, R. (eds.) 1996. Occurrence and significance of ochratoxin A in food. Food Addit. Contam. *13*, Supplement.

BLUTHGEN, A., BURT, R. and HEESCHEN, W.H. 1997. Nitrate, nitrite, nitrosamines. In *Monograph on Residues and Contaminants in Milk and Milk Products - Special Issue 9701*. (E. Hopkin, ed.) pp. 74-78, International Dairy Federation, Brussels.

BRUSSAARD, J.H., VAN DOKKUM, W., VAN DER PAAUW, C.G., DE VOS, R.H., DE KORT, W.L.A.M. and LOWIK, M.R.H. 1996. Dietary intake of food contaminants in The Netherlands (Dutch National Surveillance System). Food Addit. Contam. *13*, 561–574.

COMAS, A.P. 1982. Precocious sexual development in Puerto Rico. Lancet *i*, 1299–1300.

Commission of the European Communities Scientific Committee for Food. 1992. Report of the Scientific Committee for food on nitrate and nitrite, 26th Series. EUR 13913.

Council of the European Communities. 1981a. Council Directive 81/851/EEC on the approximation of the laws of the Member States relating to veterinary medicinal products. OJ No. *L 317*, 6.11.1981, pp. 1–17.

Council of the European Communities. 1981b. Council Directive 81/852/EEC on the approximation of the laws of the Member States relating to analytical, pharmacological and clinical standards and protocols in respect of the testing of veterinary medicinal products. OJ No. *L 317*, 6.11.1981, pp. 18–28.

DEBEUCKELAERE, W. and REMY, R. 1996. Research on the presence of antibiotic residues in meat originating from the fifteen E.U. member states. Association des Consommateurs - Test-Achats S.C., Contract No. B5-1050/95/000130.

Department of Agriculture and Food. 1997. Results of residue analysis in meat. Report No. 210/97, November 3, 2 pp. Department of Agriculture and Food, Press/Information Office, Dublin.

DE RODRIGUEZ, C.A.S. and TORO-SOLA, M.A. 1982. Anabolic steroids in meat and premature telarche. Lancet *i*, 1300.

KENNEDY, O. and O'KEEFFE, M. 1996. Generation of data on the residue status of Irish foods. Irish J. Agric. Food Res. *36*, 226.

LOIZZO, A., GATTI, G.L., MACRI, A., MORETTI, G. and ORTOLANI, E. 1984. The case of diethylstilboestrol treated veal contained in homogenized babyfoods in Italy. Methodological and toxicological aspects. Ann. Ist. Sup. Sanita. *20*, 215–220.

MACDONALD, S. and CASTLE, L. 1996. A UK survey of aflatoxins in herbs and spices and their fate during cooking. Food Addit. Contam. *13*, 121–128.

MARTINEZ-NAVARRO, J.F. 1990. Food poisoning related to consumption of illicit β-agonist in liver. Lancet *336*, 1311.

MCCRACKEN, R.J. and KENNEDY, D.G. 1997. The bioavailability of residues of the furazolidone metabolite 3-amino-2-oxazolidinone in porcine tissues and the effect of cooking upon residue concentrations. Food Addit. Contam. *14*, 507–514.

MEAH, M.N., HARRISON, N. and DAVIES, A. 1994. Nitrate and nitrite in foods and the diet. Food Addit. Contam. *11*, 519–532.

O'KEEFFE, M., EADES, J.F. and STRICKLAND, K.L. 1983. Fenthion residues in milk and milk products following treatment of dairy cows for warble-fly. J. Sci. Food Agric. *34*, 192–197.

Pesticide Control Service, Department of Agriculture, Food and Forestry. 1997. Pesticide residues in food — 1994, 1995 and 1996. pp. 96, The Stationary Office, Dublin.

PULCE, C., LAMAISON, D., KECK, G., BOSTVIRONNOIS, C., NICOLAS, J. and DESCOTES, J. 1991. Collective human food poisonings by clenbuterol residues in veal liver. Vet. Hum. Toxicol. 33, 480–481.

REMY, R. and DEBEUCKELAERE, W. 1994. Residues of growth promoting substances in meat. Association des Consommateurs - Test-Achats S.C., Contract No. B5-1050/93/006893.

ROSE, M.D., BYGRAVE, J., FARRINGTON, W.H.H. and SHEARER, G. 1996. The effect of cooking on veterinary drug residues in food: 4. oxytetracycline. Food Addit. Contam. *13*, 275–286.

ROSE, M.D., SHEARER, G. and FARRINGTON, W.H.H. 1995a. The effect of cooking on veterinary drug residues in food: 1. clenbuterol. Food Addit. Contam. *12*, 67–76.

ROSE, M.D., ARGENT, L.C., SHEARER, G. and FARRINGTON, W.H.H. 1995b. The effect of cooking on veterinary drug residues in food: 2. levamisole. Food Addit. Contam. *12*, 185–194.

ROSE, M.D., FARRINGTON, W.H.H. and SHEARER, G. 1995c. The effect of cooking on veterinary drug residues in food: 3. sulphamethazine (sulphadimidine). Food Addit. Contam. *12*, 739–750.

ROSE, M.D., SHEARER, G. and FARRINGTON, W.H.H. 1997. The effect of cooking on veterinary drug residues in food: 5. oxfendazole. Food Addit. Contam. *14*, 15–26.

SCHOENTAL, R. 1983. Precocious sexual development in Puerto Rico and oestrogenic mycotoxins (zearalenone). Lancet *i*, 537.

SCUDAMORE, K.A., HETMANSKI, M.T., CHAN, H.K. and COLLINS, S. 1997. Occurrence of mycotoxins in raw ingredients used for animal feeding stuffs in the United Kingdom in 1992. Food Addit. Contam. *14*, 157–174.

S.I. No. 218 of 1988. European Communities (Control of Oestrogenic, Androgenic, Gestagenic and Thyrostatic Substances) Regulations, 1988. The Stationary Office, Dublin.

S.I. NO. 171 of 1990. European communities (Control of Veterinary Medicinal Products and their Residues) Regulations, 1990. The Stationary Office, Dublin.

WALTERS, C.L. 1991. Nitrate and nitrite in foods. In *Nitrates and Nitrites in Food and Water*. (M.J. Hill, ed.) pp. 93–112, Ellis Horwood, London.

WALTERS, C.L. 1992. Reactions of nitrate and nitrite in foods with special reference to the determination of N-nitroso compounds. Food Addit. Contam. *9*, 441–448.

WHO. 1988. Evaluation of certain veterinary drug residues in food. *FAO/WHO Technical Report Series* 763.

WHO. 1997. The medical impact of the use of antimicrobials in food animals. *Report of WHO Meeting*, October 13-17, Berlin.

ZABIK, M.E. 1987. Pesticides and other industrial chemicals. In Toxicological Aspects of food. (K. Miller, ed.) pp. 73–102, Elsevier Applied Science, London.

CHAPTER 7

FACTORS AFFECTING THE EMERGENCE OF NEW PATHOGENS AND RESEARCH STRATEGIES LEADING TO THEIR CONTROL[1]

ARTHUR J. MILLER[2,3], JAMES L. SMITH and ROBERT L. BUCHANAN[3]

Microbial Food Safety Research Unit
Eastern Regional Research Center
Agricultural Research Service
U.S. Department of Agriculture
600 East Mermaid Lane
Wyndmoor, PA, 19038 USA

ABSTRACT

Control of foodborne emerging or reemerging microbial pathogens has proven to be difficult. Even the Hazard Analysis Critical Control Point (HACCP) approach is intended to manage known *hazards. We propose that each change occurring in the food chain — encompassing human, technological, and environmental factors — creates a new selection pressure that drives microbial adaptation and emergence potential.* Escherichia coli *O157:H7 is examined here, as a case study, to illustrate the multidimensional nature of pathogen emergence. While future emergence or reemergence events are expected, the fundamental questions of what, where, who, when, and how such events will unfold are unknown. Contingency planning can provide responses to probable hazard scenarios, with a goal of developing practical controls. Examples of potential microbial hazards and changes in the food chain are presented. Once a hazard, associated food, locale, and at-risk population are identified, critical acute research questions need to be answered. Longer term research will improve our ability to respond to the next inevitable emergence event. Such coordinated endeavors will permit rapid modification and deployment of a science-based hazard management system that will prevent or minimize human risks.*

[1] Mention of brand or firm names does not constitute an endorsement by the U.S. Department of Agriculture over others of a similar nature not mentioned.

[2] Corresponding author.

[3] Current affiliation: U.S. Food and Drug Administration, 200 "C" Street, SW, Washington, DC 20204 USA, Tel: +1-202-260-0368; email: amiller@bangate.fda.gov

INTRODUCTION

Jensen's 1942 classic *Microbiology of Meats* (Jensen 1942) lists four bacterial agents responsible for foodborne illness: *Staphylococcus aureus*, *Salmonella*, *Clostridium botulinum*, and streptococci. During the ensuing fifty-five years we have uncovered additional microbial hazards, engaging the greater capabilities of medicine, diagnostic microbiology, and epidemiology. Despite this progress, for the period 1988 to 1992, a known cause for 58.2% of reported foodborne disease outbreaks could not be determined (Bean *et al.* 1996). Emerging and reemerging pathogens undoubtedly contribute to these undiagnosed illnesses.

The U.S. Centers for Disease Control and Prevention (CDC) has defined an emerging pathogen as an infectious agent whose incidence in humans has increased dramatically within the past 20 years, or one that has the probability of increasing in the future (CDC 1994). Smith and Fratamico (1995) listed foodborne pathogens that have emerged within the past 20 years (Table 1). More recent additions include *Salmonella typhimurium* DT104 (CDC 1997a), *Cyclospora cayetanensis* (Herwaldt and Ackers 1997), *Vibrio cholerae* O139 (Albert 1994; Mooi and Bik 1997) and non-O157 serotypes of enterohemorrhagic *Escherichia coli* (Johnson *et al.* 1996).

TABLE 1.
FOODBORNE PATHOGENS THAT HAVE EMERGED WITHIN THE PAST 20 YEARS[a]

Campylobacter jejuni
Clostridium botulinum (infant botulism)
Escherichia coli O157:H7
Listeria monocytogenes
Salmonella enteritidis
Vibrio cholerae (Latin America)
Vibrio vulnificus
Yersinia enterocolitica
Norwalk and Norwalk-like viruses
Rotavirus
Cryptosporidium parvum
Giardia lamblia
Toxoplasma gondii
Bovine spongiform encephalopathy prion

[a] Smith and Fratamico 1995

The control of these hazards in foods has proven to be difficult and the routes for control have generally been chosen haphazardly. Even the Hazard Analysis Critical Control Point (HACCP) approach, which is the premier system for managing food safety hazards, is intended to manage *known* hazards. Successful hazard management is dependent upon the transformation of research-derived knowledge into practical production, processing, and food preparation practices. Considering the requirement for a preexisting and substantial body of knowledge, HACCP cannot be expected to control *unknown* hazards such as an emerging foodborne pathogen. Only the timely acquisition of critical research data can transform the hazard from the realm of the unknown to the known, and only the known can be controlled.

Thus, the aims of this paper are to classify and discuss the factors which appear to be important in the emergence or reemergence of foodborne illness and to propose a tiered approach to address research needs to control future microbial threats.

FACTORS CONTRIBUTING TO EMERGENCE OR REEMERGENCE

From the perspective of microbial ecology our sequential system of agricultural production, processing, distribution, storage, and meal preparation can be compared to a stack of micro-sieves, where each sieve selectively retains some microorganisms and lets others pass through to the next stage. In addition to hazards that are associated with raw agricultural commodities, some may be introduced during the various processing steps. Given the diversity of microorganisms on raw foods, this system reduces their numbers to a few well-adapted genera that are generally benign. Periodically, a change or failure in the control system will let a *bad bug* come through the stack.

The emergence or reemergence of an infectious disease is due to change. Table 2 lists the factors involved, and include: human (social, housing, behavioral, nutritional, demographic), technological (agricultural, medical, sanitation), environmental, and microbial adaptation elements. A few cases are elaborated to illustrate how changes in any of these factors may contribute to the emergence of new pathogens.

Agricultural Practice Changes

(1) Extensive antibiotic use in animals has allegedly led to the emergence of a multidrug-resistant *S. typhimurium*, Designation Type (DT) 104 (Meslin 1997). In Europe and North America, the organism is quickly becoming the dominant phage-type of this *Salmonella* serovar. Its resistance genes reside chromosomally, which indicates that resistance is likely to be retained even in the absence of antibiotics. It is unclear if the resistance genes form a single block on the chromosome, i.e., a resistance island (Hecker *et al.* 1997), or if they are inserted randomly into the chromosome. Furthermore, it is unknown if these genes are associated with pathogenicity islands, which

have been described in *Salmonella* (Groisman and Ochman 1997). While we know that the organism exhibits enhanced virulence, compared to other salmonellae, we have little information about its survival and growth potential in food systems (Humphrey 1997). Transmission can occur when animals are raised in close proximity, since it is possible to isolate the drug-resistant pathogen from animals not subjected to antibiotic treatment (Meslin 1997). As with most salmonellae, humans can be infected via animal contact or by ingesting raw or undercooked meats from animals and poultry infected with the organism. The use of DT104-containing manures on crop lands also may contaminate vegetable crops.

(2) Infection of the oviduct of laying hens with *Salmonella enteritidis* has led to outbreaks of human salmonellosis involving shell eggs (Humphrey 1994; St. Louis *et al.* 1988). Consumers have generally assumed that grade A shell eggs are safe and that egg contents are bacteria-free. The strains of *S. enteritidis* involved in these outbreaks have been shown to be invasive for chickens and the invasive strains causing foodborne outbreaks are closely related (Hinton *et al.* 1990; Stanley *et al.* 1992). Improper storage of grade A eggs allowing the growth of *S. enteritidis* (Bradshaw *et al.* 1990) combined with consumer preference for undercooked eggs or products containing raw eggs (Klontz *et al.* 1995; Mishu *et al.* 1991) are factors involved in outbreaks. Various poultry raising practices and industrialization of poultry breeding, poultry rearing, egg production and egg distribution have probably also contributed to the emergence and persistence of *S. enteritidis* (Smith and Fratamico 1995).

Technology Changes

(1) Bovine spongiform encephalopathy (BSE) emerged as an infectious agent, mainly from adult dairy cattle in the United Kingdom. The evidence indicates that this prion-derived disease was a result of feeding cattle, meat and bone meal (MBM; derived from dead ruminants, such as sheep, and slaughter house by-products, infected with scrapie) as a protein supplement (Nathanson 1997). Reduction of temperature used in heat treatment and elimination of solvent extraction of animal tissue during MBM processing apparently led to a failure to inactivate the BSE prion and allowed its introduction into the cattle population (Collee and Bradley 1997; Nathanson 1997). The ban on the use of MBM has led to a steady decline in the number of BSE infected cattle in the United Kingdom (Collee and Bradley 1997). Will *et al.* (1996) has suggested that ingesting BSE-containing meat may lead to Creutzfeldt-Jakob disease in humans, but the evidence is tenuous.

TABLE 2.
FACTORS INVOLVED IN EMERGENCE/RE-EMERGENCE OF PATHOGENS[a]

Factor	Examples
Social	Economic impoverishment War Civil conflict or political upheaval Population demographics (growth or migration) Urbanization (decay, crowding)
Technological	Changes in medical technology (medical devices, immunosuppressive drugs) Industrialized food production and processing (consolidation, preservation technologies) Globalization of food supplies (Imports, uneducated workers)
Health care and public health infra-structure	Increased organ and tissue transplantation Antibiotic use Increased use of nursing homes for the elderly Reduction or elimination of disease prevention programs Inadequate infectious disease surveillance Insufficient numbers of trained public health personnel Inadequate treatment of potable water supplies and sewage
Demographics	Increase in number of immigrants Increase in number of elderly individuals Increase in number of immunocompromised individuals (malnourished, medically immunosuppressed, diseased, nursing home residents, organ transplant patients)
Human behavior	Changes in sexual behavior Increased use of recreational drugs (intravenous) Changes in diet (new foods, fewer meals eaten at home) Shift of women from home to workplace Increased use of child day care facilities (single parents or dual income families) Increase in number of pets (domestic and exotic) Increased international business travel and tourism Decrease in breast feeding
Environmental	Deforestation and/or reforestation Changes in water ecosystems (building of dams, irrigation) Climate (flooding or drought conditions, global warming) Famine Earthquakes Heat waves or cold spells Algae blooms
Microbial adaptation	Increase in or gaining of virulence factors and/or toxin production Development of drug resistance Microorganisms as cofactors in chronic diseases (toxoplasmosis in AIDS patients) Microorganisms crossing species barriers Introduction of pathogens into new geographic areas Ability to adapt to new environmental conditions
Vectors	Introduction to new geographic areas (climate changes; human migration) Development of resistance to pesticides Change in land or water ecology

a) Centers for Disease Control and Prevention 1994; Hedberg *et al.* 1994; Lederberg *et al.* 1992; Levine and Levine 1994; Smith and Fratamico 1995

(2) The emergence of *Listeria monocytogenes* as a major foodborne pathogen is directly related to increased use of long-term cold storage of foods. The psychrotrophic nature of *L. monocytogenes* allows its growth at refrigeration temperatures (Smith and Fratamico 1995). The predilection of the organism for immunocompromised individuals makes *L. monocytogenes* a particularly dangerous foodborne pathogen to a major segment of the population (Schuchat *et al.* 1991).

Public Health Policy Change

In order to reduce cancer risks, officials in Peru eliminated chlorination of drinking water (Anderson 1991). This decision resulted in a cholera epidemic occurring throughout much of Latin America. The poor infrastructure of potable water distribution and sewage disposal systems has made eradication of epidemic cholera in Latin America difficult (Swerdlow *et al.* 1992). The use of contaminated water to prepare food as well as preparation of food by infected food handlers has led to unsafe foods.

Microbial Adaptation

El Tor serotype O1 strains have been responsible for epidemic cholera in Asia, Africa and South America. Interestingly, in 1992, epidemic cholera due to serotype O139 *V. cholerae* emerged and has spread through southeast Asia (Albert 1994). A toxin-producing *V. cholerae* probably acquired the O139 antigen by horizontal gene transfer; the emergence of the new cholera toxin-producing serotype may have been facilitated by naturally acquired immunity to the O1 serotype (Mooi and Bik 1997). What is even more interesting, a new clone of El Tor O1 has displaced O139 as the cholera-producing organism in Calcutta. This new clone has a different ribotype from El Tor O1 present before the O139 outbreaks (Sharma *et al.* 1997). Faruque *et al.* (1997) have presented evidence that a new ribotype of Bengal O139 has recently appeared in Bangladesh. Cycling of successive ribotypes of O1 El Tor with O139 may well be the pattern of future cholera outbreaks in Asia.

The ability for bacteria to adapt to changes in their environment cannot be overemphasized. For many enteric bacteria, a single DNA change can convert a microorganism into a pathogen (Groisman and Ochman 1997). Moreover, as described below for *E. coli* O157:H7, hypermutable genetic sequences exist in bacteria, termed contingency loci, to facilitate rapid diversification (Deitsch *et al.* 1997). Indeed, for some pathogenic bacteria, it has been shown that an entire population of infecting organisms can be derived from a single clone (Moxon and Murphy 1978). Thus, in our efforts to keep food safe by developing adequate preservation systems, we are confronted with remarkably adaptable bacterial antagonists.

ESCHERICHIA COLI O157:H7 AS A MODEL FOR THE EMERGENCE OF A FOODBORNE PATHOGEN

While a single change factor is frequently the direct cause of an outbreak by a new pathogen, a series of contributing underlying events have usually occurred prior to emergence in the human population. The emergence of *E. coli* O157:H7 as a major foodborne pathogen can provide insights to understand the multidimensional nature of emergence. For example, while undercooking was the primary factor contributing to beefburger outbreaks, the accumulation of virulence factors by the bacterium, shifts in livestock raising techniques, consolidation of the slaughter and processing segments of the industry, and modifications in human eating habits (Armstrong *et al.* 1996) also needed to occur. Each of these underlying components can be expanded.

Evolution of *E. coli* O157:H7 Pathogenicity

Clinical isolates from hemorrhagic colitis or HUS patients belong to a single genetic clonal group (Whittam *et al.* 1988). These strains are unrelated to those of the O157 serogroup, that lack the H7 antigen (Whittam and Wilson 1988). Instead, O157:H7 is genetically related to O55:H7 strains. (Whittam *et al.* 1993). Whittam *et al.* (1993) visualized the origin of O157:H7 as follows:

> A O55:H7-like ancestor with the ability to cause disease via the attaching-effacing mechanism acquired the capability for producing Shiga-like toxin and adhesins via horizontal genetic transfer from other pathogens and by recombination. Acquisition of a new serogroup antigen (O157) led to the appearance of a new, highly virulent organism — *E. coli* O157:H7.

The initial localization sites for *E. coli* O157:H7 in cattle are the fore-stomachs where fermentation takes place (Doyle *et al.* 1997). Thus, the necessity to survive the acidic gastric environment probably created a selective pressure for *E. coli* O157:H7 to acquire acid tolerance (Foster 1995; Archer 1996). As a consequence, the pathogen can grow and/or survive in acidic foods (Conner and Kotrola 1995; Diez-Gonzalez and Russell 1997; Waterman and Small 1996). The ability to acquire such virulence genes may result from demonstrated increased mutation rates and enhanced recombination abilities (Moxon *et al.* 1994; LeClerc *et al.* 1996).

Hypermutability of *E. coli* O157:H7 suggests that the organism may acquire new factors that will render it even more virulent. In addition, Baur *et al.*

(1996) reported that *E. coli* became maximally competent for genetic transformation in freshwater environments when the bacterium was exposed to ≥2 mM Ca^{2+}, as temperatures increased from 10 to 20C. In the broad sense, these results and those of Pupo *et al.* (1997) suggest that any *E. coli* strain which acquires virulence factors may give rise to a pathogenic type.

Changes in the Cattle Industry

There is likely a close relationship between animal management practices and the presence of *E. coli* O157:H7 (Armstrong *et al.* 1996; Hancock *et al.* 1997a,b). While *E. coli* O157:H7 was isolated from sheep, goats, horses, dogs, deer and wild birds feces (Chalmers *et al.* 1997; Keene *et al.* 1997; Kudva *et al.* 1997; Wallace *et al.* 1997), beef and dairy cattle appear to be the main reservoir in the United States. Changes in the cattle industry may have influenced emergence or persistence of *E. coli* O157:H7. For example, in the United States, there are fewer feedlots now with capacity of <1000 head, and more with a capacity of ≥16,000 cattle. In addition, feedlot preponderance has changed location from the upper midwestern states to the warmer lower midwestern states (Armstrong *et al.* 1996). Similarly, the dairy industry has shifted to fewer and larger facilities, with a large share of milk production shifted to western and southwestern states from northeastern and upper midwestern states (Armstrong *et al.* 1996). The concentration of larger numbers of animals in fewer facilities, combined with shifts to warmer locations, has perhaps led to increased prevalence of *E. coli* O157:H7 in slaughter cattle. Contributing factors include confinement and crowding, feed deprivation and trucking stresses associated with transport to slaughter. Such factors allow cattle to shed *E. coli* O157:H7 in feces (Rasmussen *et al.* 1993).

E. coli O157:H7 survives for long periods in animal fecal slurries (Kudva *et al.* 1995) which suggests that such manures could provide a source of contamination for cattle; however, Hancock *et al.* (1997a) demonstrated that prevalence of the pathogen in dairy herds was not correlated with the use of manure slurries on cattle forage crop land or pasture. Cattle manure on farmland is the probable source for the presence of *E. coli* O157:H7 in wild bird (mostly gulls) feces (Wallace *et al.* 1997). Thus, wild birds could be the vector for the transfer of the pathogen to cattle and other ruminants.

Changes in Cattle Slaughtering, Meat Processing and Meat Distribution

In the slaughterhouse, carcasses can become contaminated with feces containing the pathogen. Slaughter facilities have decreased in number, in the U.S., but those remaining have grown larger. These large facilities slaughter animals from multi-state regions, which involves stressful long-term trucking, feed deprivation, and stressful crowding. Stressful conditions can stimulate pathogen excretion, increasing potential for carcass contamination during slaughter. Large processing and boning facilities take chilled carcasses and produce boned beef and trimmings that are co-mingled with meat from many carcasses. In turn, beef-grinding operations receive different types of raw material from multiple suppliers, further compounding the problem. Boneless beef and trimmings are blended without trace-back capabilities, if a problem should arise. The recent Hudson Food beefburger recall brought to light the common industrial practice of mixing the previous day's unused blends with today's product. Beef patties are shipped to food distribution centers which purvey the patties to food markets and to food service establishments (Armstrong *et al.* 1996; Levine and Levine 1994).

The increased industrialization of animal husbandry, slaughter, food processing and food distribution allows the consumer to buy foods readily and at reasonable prices. However, if a food is contaminated, the business concentration effect results in distribution of that pathogen to larger segments of the consuming population, which magnifies their potential risk (Smith and Fratamico 1995).

Changes in the Eating Habits of Consumers

Approximately half of all American's meals are eaten away from home, mostly in restaurants (Jensen and Unnevehr 1995); control over food preparation is rapidly being lost, perhaps with heightened risks. In addition, some consumers dislike the idea of pasteurization or heat treatment of certain foods. Thus, consumers can become infected with *E. coli* O157:H7 after consumption of unpasteurized apple cider (Besser *et al.* 1993; CDC 1997b) or apple juice (CDC 1996) or fermented but uncooked salami (CDC 1995; Tilden *et al.* 1996). Even when products are cooked there is frequently a preference for minimal cooking. For example, approximately 25% of respondents in a United States survey expressed a preference for rare or medium-cooked hamburgers (Klontz *et al.* 1995). Unlike other beef cuts where microbial contamination is confined to the surface, ground meat has microorganisms distributed throughout the product. In the preparation of a rare or medium steak, the cooking process destroys the surface organisms, but rare or medium-cooked hamburger will still contain a substantial microbial population. Since the infectious dose of *E. coli* O157:H7 is very low, the person who prefers rare or medium-cooked hamburgers is at risk (Armstrong *et al.* 1996; Tilden *et al.* 1996).

E. coli O157:H7 has probably emerged several times in the past, but its success as a pathogen persisted only when the changes discussed above occurred. It is critical to learn what factors can cause pathogens to emerge, and, attempt to predict a potential emergence.

ANTICIPATING THE NEXT EMERGING PATHOGEN

While future emergence or reemergence events can be expected, the complex questions of what, where, who, when, and how such events will unfold are unknown. The challenge becomes to plan for a microbial threat. Military contingency planning may be applied to this problem. This approach to preventing or minimizing consequences of potential outbreaks has four components: intelligence, personnel and facilities, rapid response, and strategic planning. Each is discussed below.

Intelligence consists of information gathering activities, in this case to permit an emergence to be identified. In the United States, the CDC serves as a clearinghouse for this activity, in direct cooperation with state public health agencies; however, CDC's surveillance activities are largely domestic, whereas an effective intelligence system for foodborne disease of necessity must be worldwide. Other potential sources of information include: The World Health Organization, other sovereign governments, the U.S. military's international network of laboratory and medical investigators, the medical and scientific literature, and the Internet. Intelligence gathering must include an awareness of changes and advances in food technology, agricultural practices and conditions, veterinary medicine, environmental and water microbiology, consumer trends, and general socioeconomic conditions. This information must be analyzed by experts to determine the potential impact on public health.

The second component of contingency planning is to ensure the availability of personnel and facilities to quickly characterize a new biological agent, then to develop control strategies. The broad range of capabilities and resources needed to deal with all contingencies will unlikely reside in a single organization. One approach is to establish "reserve" groups of subject-matter experts from various organizations that could coordinately mobilize as needed. This requires centralized planning, periodic drills, and inter-organizational cooperation to ensure that needed expertises and facilities are maintained.

The third component of contingency planning is rapid resource mobilization. Currently, the focus of rapid response efforts has been directed largely on the diagnosis of illness, identification of new agents, and the recall of suspect food. These are key initial steps; however, the initiation of critical research to prevent another occurrence of the emerging pathogen has been handled typically in a much less organized and timely manner, and should commence at this stage of response.

The fourth component, strategic planning, should be the first step to be conducted. Strategic planning involves simulating "what we would do if" scenarios, especially planning appropriate responses. This has received little attention in relation to emerging foodborne pathogens. This process relies on "futurist thinking" to consider changes in society, economics, technology, agriculture, medicine, international trade, etc. in view of their likely impact on microbiological safety of the food supply. A broad view is needed since root causes of most disease emergences are general events or trends in society. Strategic planning is undertaken with the realization that the probability of a specific "what - if" scenario occurring is low, but the probability that one of many alternatives will occur is high.

FORECAST FOR PATHOGEN EMERGENCE

Nearly all microbial foodborne disease stems from consumption of either raw, undercooked, temperature abused, or cross-contaminated products, as the immediate cause (Bryan 1988). Thus, if these shortcomings were remedied, few outbreaks would occur. Yet, in the U.S., government agencies and the food industry have accepted as a challenge the reduction or elimination of the microbial hazards from the food supply. This is best demonstrated by the endorsement of HACCP by organizations, such as the American Meat Institute, the USDA Pathogen Reduction/HACCP rule, and, most recently, by the announcement of the Food Safety Initiative by President Clinton. These measures, however, primarily address known hazards. The emerging hazards remain in the realm of the unknown.

We can predict that new pathogens will emerge. We know they will emerge from either a failure of a traditional safeguard or from a change that creates an organism adapted to overcome the traditional safeguard. In this section, we offer some "intelligence" by providing examples of newer microbial hazards seen in the medical or veterinary community and of global trends in human demands, technology and trade that could affect food safety.

Pathogens with Potential for Emergence

Prion-Induced Variant Creutzfeldt-Jakob Disease. New variant Creutzfeldt-Jakob disease (nvCJD) has occurred in the United Kingdom and Europe. Unlike CJD, nvCJD presents with a pathology similar to BSE and thus this raised fears that the eating of BSE-infected meats may lead to nvCJD (Will *et al.* 1996). A disease similar to nvCJD has been induced in macaques by intracerebral inoculation of tissue from BSE-infected cattle (Lasmézas *et al.* 1996). However, *in vitro* experimental results suggest that transmission of the infectious agent of BSE and scrapie to humans is quite low (Raymond *et al.* 1997). Lantos *et al.* (1997) have demonstrated that there are many similarities between nvCJD and kuru. Kuru is a transmissible spongiform encephalopathy (TSE) associated with cannibalism. It is possible that the similarities in phenotypic presentation of kuru and nvCJD, both clinically and neuropathologically, reflect a common route of infection — oral ingestion of prion-infected tissue which leads to disease. Since TSEs develop so slowly, it may be difficult to prove that an oral route of infection can lead to nvCJD.

If nvCJD arises from BSE ingestion, the factors that led to the emergence of nvCJD have been changed, i.e., elimination of feeding MBM derived from ruminants, destruction of BSE-infected cattle, elimination of ruminant central nervous tissue in meats. Since nvCJD probably has a long incubation period, 10-15 years, in humans, there may be an increase in nvCJD for the next few years before the disease disappears.

Viruses. It is certain that a portion of the outbreaks with unknown etiology are due to foodborne viruses. As virus detection technology improves, especially by the use of DNA-probes, more foodborne viruses will be recognized. It is probable that many of the factors that led to the emergence of *E. coli* O157:H7 also are important in viral emergence. Many of the foodborne viruses are also waterborne and the aging of potable water infrastructure will play a role in virus emergence.

Bacteria.

Citrobacter freundii. C. freundii is an intestinal commensal bacterium of humans and animals, which is present in water, sewage, soil and foods (Stiles 1989). The microorganism is an opportunistic pathogen in immunocompromised individuals (Lipsky *et al.* 1980; Samonis *et al.* 1991). Karasawa *et al.* (1990) found that *C. freundii* isolated from an infant with diarrhea produced a heat-labile toxin similar to cholera toxin and *E. coli* heat-labile toxin. Strains of *C. freundii* isolated from diarrheic children were shown to produce heat-stable toxin similar to that produced by enterotoxigenic *E. coli* (Guarino *et al.* 1987, 1989). Shiga-like toxin (SLT) II but not SLT I has been found in *C. freundii* strains isolated from diarrheic patients (Schmidt *et al.* 1993). Interestingly, a foodborne outbreak was reported by Tschäpe *et al.* (1995) in which SLT-II producing *C. freundii* were isolated from stools of patients with severe gastroenteritis and hemolytic uremic syndrome. Since *C. freundii* has the ability to produce and/or acquire a number of toxins, it seems likely that the organism could emerge as an important foodborne pathogen in the future. In the outbreak described by Tschäpe *et al.* (1995), green butter (parsley in butter) was the causative food. The parsley was grown organically in a garden fertilized with pig manure. SLT-II-producing *E. coli* O139 was isolated from the parsley in addition to *Citrobacter*. It is probable that the toxin-producing gene was transferred from *E. coli* to *Citrobacter*. With the increasing demand for organically grown food, more such outbreaks may occur unless the animal manures are sterilized to prevent transfer of toxin genes from one species to another.

Arcobacter butzleri. *A. butzleri* is present in a variety of foods including poultry, beef and pork (de Boer *et al.* 1996; Zanetti *et al.* 1996). The organism has been isolated from the feces of diarrheic animals and humans (Anderson *et al.* 1993; Kiehlbach *et al.* 1991). *A. butzleri* has been associated with severe diarrhea in immunocompromised individuals (Lerner *et al.* 1994) and bacteremia in a neonate (On *et al.* 1995). Essentially nothing is known about virulence factors in *A. butzleri*; however, Musmanno *et al.* (1997) examined 18 river isolates for virulence factors. Seventeen strains produced a cytotoxin active against Vero cells with production of cell rounding and nuclear pyknosis. One strain had cytotonic activity against CHO cells with production of cell elongation; the strain also was adherent to intestine 407 cells. Cytolethal distending effects or invasion was not observed for any of the 18 strains (Musmanno *et al.* 1997). Future studies should concentrate on virulence factors and the disease-inducing ability of *A. butzleri*. So little is known about *Arcobacter*, it is difficult to know what may be involved in its potential emergence. It is probable that many of the factors involved in the emergence of *E. coli* O157:H7 will be involved in the emergence of *Arcobacter*.

Salmonella. The recent identification of sub-populations of *S. enteriditus* PT4 (Humphrey *et al.* 1995) and *S. typhimurium* DT104 (Humphrey 1997) exhibiting enhanced survival characteristics suggests that this genus may be acquiring new survival genes. If true, this may necessitate reevaluating past practices, which were based on *Salmonella* inactivation.

Parasites. The demand for a year round supply of fresh produce creates opportunities for equatorial and Southern hemisphere countries that are fruit and vegetable producers. Similar to the emergence of *Cyclospora* in North America, we will in all likelihood see other parasites. The poor potable water infrastructure of developing countries (similar to that seen in Peru in the South American cholera outbreak) will ensure that even more parasites will emerge. As long as the water infrastructure of the developed nations remains intact, secondary cases of emerging parasites will be rare.

Human, Technology, and Environmental Factors

Trends in human demographics and consumer demands, technological breakthroughs, and the resultant infrastructure and land or water use practices, undoubtedly will create new niches for microbial hazards to emerge. The growing demand for a year-round supply of fresh foods, is offered as an example. The technology to satisfy this demand may be near, as FastShip container vessels — using water jet or gas turbine engines and alternative hull design — hold promise to cut transoceanic shipping time by nearly half (Giles

1997). Coupled with highly efficient loading and unloading systems, and land-based transportation systems keeping to tight schedules, massive quantities of fresh products will travel to foreign markets at high speed. This increased product availability, will heighten consumer demand, which will stimulate further international commerce in fresh fruits, vegetables, and seafood. One consequence may be the rapid dissemination of previously localized infectious organisms carried on contaminated products. Another consequence may be the spread of human pathogens from biofilms on the hull, and the bilge water carried within ships. As a case-in-point, the Peru *Vibrio* pandemic was disseminated by the dumping of *V. cholerae* laden bilge water into foreign harbors. Globalization of fresh food markets will undoubtedly create pressures to increase production, which, if implemented without considering potential public health effects, may lead to increased health risks. For example, intensive aquaculture, integration of hydroponics with aquaculture waste streams, and uncontrolled manuring of crop lands may offer attractive approaches to boost product yields, but also create new opportunities for pathogen emergence. Other trends, with health implications, include: consumer demand for nontraditional foods, without additional safety education; shipment of food during seasonal contamination cycles; and the demand for preservative-free foods. Any or all of these may result in an outbreak of foodborne illness from a heretofore unknown organism, or an old pest may reemerge.

TWO-TIERED APPROACH TO ADDRESSING RESEARCH NEEDS

Buchanan (1997) described two distinct classes of research needs on emerging pathogens, based on time constraints. Acute research needs provide knowledge and technology to control the emerging pathogen. It is specific to the microorganism and food and must be accomplished swiftly. This research is generally applied, though basic research may overcome deficiencies in knowledge, if little information exists. General areas include: diagnostics, food vehicles, contamination sources, pathogen growth and survival characteristics, microbial ecology, virulence characteristics, and at-risk human populations. In short, any data necessary to prevent a reoccurrence of the disease or to modify current HACCP, good production, or good manufacturing practices should be classified as an acute research need.

Buchanan (1997) described three components of longer term research associated with emerging pathogens. The first area is research to find improvements or alternatives to detect and control the emerging pathogen. The second area is research to reduce the response time between the emergence of a pathogen and its initial control. The third area is research that identifies factors that will allow new microbial threats to be anticipated.

WARS AVOIDED; BATTLES WON

Recent events demonstrate that we have been successful in identifying some potential hazards and reacting quickly to avoid or minimize adverse health consequences. Three examples are described.

Sous Vide

Precooked modified atmosphere or vacuum-packaged refrigerated entrees, introduced during the 1980's, are a potentially high risk food class that has not resulted in foodborne illness. Products, such as *sous vide,* are minimally pasteurized, lack conventional preservatives, and are maintained at refrigerated temperatures under an oxygen-free atmosphere. Potential hazards include the outgrowth of spores of nonproteolytic *Clostridium botulinum*, which can germinate at 3.3C, and the absence of microbial competition, primarily lactic acid organisms, to acidify a temperature-abused product, and inhibit pathogen growth. These concerns have been overcome by formulating acidified sauces which serve in the same role as the lactic acid organisms.

Fresh Mushrooms

Soon after oxygen barrier over-wraps were introduced into the U.S. market to extend the shelf life of fresh mushrooms, it was recognized that spores of *Clostridium botulinum* which are frequently associated with the product, could germinate and produce neurotoxin, after the aerobic microflora consumed residual oxygen. The problem was avoided by introducing a sufficient number of holes in the film to prevent anaerobic conditions from forming.

Listeria monocytogenes

Once it was recognized as a foodborne pathogen, and control measures were introduced, the annual incidence of human illness in the U.S. decreased by nearly 50% (Tappero *et al.* 1995). The record thus demonstrates that food safety can be ensured if proper controls are implemented.

CONCLUSIONS

For every change we impose on the food chain, we create a new selection pressure that increases the probability that a pathogen will emerge or reemerge. Yet, it is obvious to anyone associated with the food industry that change is unavoidable. Therefore, emergence of new or old pathogens can be expected to occur. When possible, we need to predict potential hazards and establish proactive control measures. When a pathogen emerges, we need to minimize its human health impact by quickly establishing controls. If the technology or knowledge is lacking, a research effort is warranted. The overall goal needs to be hazard management throughout production, processing, distribution, and final food preparation.

REFERENCES

ALBERT, M.J. 1994. *Vibrio cholerae* O139 Bengal. J. Clin. Microbiol. *32*, 2345–2349.

ANDERSON, C. 1991. Cholera epidemic traced to risk miscalculation. Nature *354*, 255.

ANDERSON, K.F. *et al.* 1993 *Arcobacter (Campylobacter) butzleri*-associated diarrheal illness in a nonhuman primate population. Infect. Immun. *61*, 2220–2223.

ARCHER, D.L. 1996 Preservation microbiology and safety: Evidence that stress enhances virulence and triggers adaptive mutations. Trends Food Sci. Technol. *7*, 91–95.

ARMSTRONG, G.L., HOLLINGSWORTH, J. and MORRIS, J.G. 1996. Emerging foodborne pathogens: *Escherichia coli* O157:H7 as a model of entry of a new pathogen into the food supply of the developed world. Epidemiol. Rev. *18*, 29–51.

BAUR, B., HANSELMAN, K., SCHLIMME, W. and JENNI, B. 1996. Genetic transformation in freshwater: *Escherichia coli* is able to develop natural competence. Appl. Environ. Microbiol. *62*, 3673–3678.

BEAN, N.H., GOULDING, J.S., LAO, C. and ANGULO, F.J. 1996. Surveillance for foodborne-disease outbreaks – United States, 1988-1992. Morb. Mort. Weekly Rept. *45* (No. SS-5), 16–20.

BESSER, R.E. *et al.* 1993. An outbreak of diarrhea and hemolytic uremic syndrome from *Escherichia coli* O157:H7 in fresh-pressed apple cider. J. Am. Med. Assoc. *269*, 2217–2220.

BRADSHAW, J.G., SHAH, D.B., FORNEY, E. and MADDEN, J.M. 1990. Growth of *Salmonella enteritidis* in yolk of shell eggs from normal and seropositive hens. J. Food Prot. *53*, 1033–1036.

BRYAN, F.L. 1988. Risks of practices, procedures and processes that lead to outbreaks of foodborne diseases. J. Food Protect. *51*, 663–673.

BUCHANAN, R.L. 1997. Research needs for identifying and controlling emerging foodborne pathogens. Emerging Infect. Dis. *3*, 517–521.

CDC 1994. Addressing Emerging Infectious Disease Threats: A Prevention Strategy for the United States. U.S. Dept. Health and Human Services, Public Health Service, Atlanta, GA, USA.

CDC 1995. *Escherichia coli* O157:H7 outbreak linked to commercially distributed dry-cured salami - Washington and California, 1994. Morb. Mort. Weekly Rept. *44*, 157–160.

CDC 1996. Outbreaks of *Escherichia coli* O157:H7 infections associated with drinking unpasteurized apple juice – British Columbia, California, Colorado, and Washington, October 1996. Morb. Mort. Weekly Rept. *45*, 975.

CDC 1997a. Multidrug-resistant *Salmonella* serotype typhimurium — United States, 1996. Morb. Mort. Weekly Rept. *46*, 308–310.

CDC 1997b. Outbreaks of *Escherichia coli* O157:H7 infection and cryptosporidiosis associated with drinking unpasteurized apple cider - Connecticut and New York, October 1996. Morb. Mort. Weekly Rept. *46*, 4–8.

CHALMERS, R.M. *et al.* 1997. Vero-cytotoxin-producing *Escherichia coli* O157 in a farmer handling horses. Lancet *349*, 1816.

COLLEE, J.G. and BRADLEY, R. 1997. BSE: a decade on – part 1. Lancet *349*, 636–641.

CONNER, D.E. and KOTROLA, J.S. 1995. Growth and survival of *Escherichia coli* O157:H7 under acidic conditions. Appl. Environ. Microbiol. *61*, 382–385.

de BOER, E. *et al.* 1996. A selective medium for the isolation of *Arcobacter* from meats. Lett. Appl. Microbiol. *23*, 64–66.

DEITSCH, K.W., MOXON, E.R. and WELLEMS, T.E. 1997. Shared themes of antigenic variation and virulence in bacterial, protozoal, and fungal infections. Microbiol. Mol. Biol. Rev. *61*, 281–293.

DIEZ-GONZALEZ, F. and RUSSELL, J.B. 1997. The ability of *Escherichia coli* O157:H7 to decrease its intracellular pH and resist toxicity of acetic acid. Microbiology *143*, 1175–1180.

DOYLE, M.P., ZHAO, T., MENG, T. and ZHAO, S. 1997. *Escherichia coli* O157:H7, In *Food Microbiology: Fundamentals and Frontiers*, (M.P. Doyle, L.R. Beuchat and T.J. Montville, eds.) pp. 171–191, ASM Press, Washington, DC.

FARUQUE, S.M. *et al.*. 1997. Molecular analysis of toxigenic *Vibrio cholerae* O139 Bengal strains isolated in Bangladesh between 1993 and 1996: evidence for emergence of a new clone of the Bengal vibrios. J. Clin. Microbiol. *35*, 2299–2306.

FOSTER, J.W. 1995. Low pH adaptation and the acid tolerance response of *Salmonella typhimurium*. Critical Rev Microbiol. *21*, 215–237.

GILES, D.L. 1997 Faster ships for the future. Sci. Am. *227*(4), 126–131.

GROISMAN, E.A. and OCHMAN, H. 1997. How *Salmonella* became a pathogen. Trends in Microbiol. *5*, 343–349.

GUARINO, A. *et al.* 1987. Production of *Escherichia coli* STa-like heat-stable enterotoxin by *Citrobacter freundii* isolated from humans. J. Clin. Microbiol. *25*, 110–114.

GUARINO, A., GIANNELLA, R. and THOMPSON, M.R. 1989. *Citrobacter freundii* produces an 18-amino-acid heat-stable enterotoxin identical to the 18-amino-acid *Escherichia coli* heat-stable enterotoxin (ST Ia). Infect. Immun. *57*, 649–652.

HANCOCK, D.D., *et al.* 1997a. Effects of farm manure-handling practices on *Escherichia coli* O157 prevalence in cattle. J. Food Prot. *60*, 363–366.

HANCOCK, D.D. *et al.* 1997b. Epidemiology of *Escherichia coli* O157 in feedlot cattle. J. Food Prot. *60*, 462–465.

HECKER, J., BLUM-OEHLER, G., MUHLDORFER, I. and TSCHÄPE, H. 1997. Pathogenicity islands of virulent bacteria: structure, function and impact on microbial evolution. Molec. Microbiol. *23*, 1089–1097.

HEDBERG, C.W., MACDONALD, K.L. and OSTERHOLM, M.T. 1994. Changing epidemiology of food-borne disease: A Minnesota perspective. Clin. Infect. Dis. *18*, 671–682.

HERWALDT, B.L. and ACKERS, M.-L. 1997. An outbreak in 1996 of cyclosporiasis associated with imported raspberries. N. Engl. J. Med. *336*, 1548–1556.

HINTON, M., THRELFALL, E.J. and ROWE, B. 1990. The invasive potential of *Salmonella enteritidis* phage types for young chickens. Lett. Appl. Microbiol. *10*, 237–239.

HUMPHREY, T.J. 1994. Contamination of egg shell and contents with *Salmonella enteritidis*: a review. Intl. J. Food Microbiol. *21*, 31–40.

HUMPHREY, T.J. 1997. Personal communication.

HUMPHREY, T.J., SLATER, E., MCALPINE, K., ROWBURY, R.J. and GILBERT, R.J. 1995 *Salmonella enteritidis* phage type 4 isolates more tolerant of heat, acid, or hydrogen peroxide also survive longer on surfaces. Appl. Environ. Microbiol *61*, 3161–3164.

JENSEN, L.B. 1942. *Microbiology of Meats*, Garrard Press, Champaign.

JENSEN, H. and UNNEVEHR, L. 1995. The economics of regulation and information related to foodborne microbial pathogens, In *Tracking Foodborne Pathogens from Farm to Table: Data Needs to Evaluate Control Options, U.S.D.A, Economic Research Service, Food and Consumer Economics Division*. (T. Roberts, H. Jensen and L. Unnevehr, eds.) pp. 125–133 Misc. Pub. #1532.

JOHNSON, R.P. *et al.* 1996. Growing concerns and recent outbreaks involving non-0157:H7 serotypes of verotoxigenic *Escherichia coli*. J. Food Prot. *59*, 1112–1122.

KARASAWA, T., ITO, H., TSUKAMOTO, T., NISHIBUCHI, M. and TAKEDA, Y. 1990. Molecular genetic analysis of a factor produced by *Citrobacter freundii* which immunologically cross-reacted with cholera toxin (CT) and heat-labile enterotoxin (LTh). Jpn. J. Med. Sci. Biol. *43*, 247–248.

KEENE, W.E. *et al.* 1997. An outbreak of *Escherichia coli* O157:H7 infections traced to jerky made from deer meat. J. Am. Med. Assoc. *277*, 1229–1231.

KIEHLBACH, J.A. *et al.* 1991. *Campylobacter butzleri* sp. nov. isolated from humans and animals with diarrheal illness. J. Clin. Microbiol. *29*, 376–385.

KLONTZ, K.C., TIMBO, B., FEIN, S. and LEVY, A. 1995. Prevalence of selected food consumption and preparation behaviors associated with increased risks of food-borne disease. J. Food Prot. *58*, 927–930.

KUDVA, I.T., HATFIELD, P.G. and HOVDE, C.J. 1995. Effect of diet on the shedding of *Escherichia coli* O157:H7 in a sheep model. Appl. Environ. Microbiol. *61*, 1363–1370.

KUDVA, I.T., HATFIELD, P.G. and HOVDE, C.J. 1997. Characterization of *Escherichia coli* O157:H7 and other Shiga toxin-producing *E. coli* serotypes isolated from sheep. J. Clin. Microbiol. *35*, 892–899.

LANTOS, P.L. *et al.* 1997. Is the neuropathology of new variant Creutzfeldt-Jakob disease and kuru similar? Lancet *350*, 187–188.

LASMÉZAS, C.I. *et al.* 1996. BSE transmission to macaques. Nature *381*, 743–744.

LECLERC, J.E., LI, B., PAYNE, W.L. and CEBULA, T.A. 1996. High mutation frequencies among *Escherichia coli* and *Salmonella* pathogens. Science *274*, 1208–1211.

LEDERBERG, J., SHOPE, R.E. and OAKS, S.C. (eds.) 1992. *Emerging Infections: Microbial Threats to Health in the United States*, National Academy Press, Washington, DC.

LERNER, J., BRUMBERGER, V. and PREAC-MURSIC, V. 1994. Severe diarrhea associated with *Arcobacter butzleri*. Eur. J. Clin. Microbiol. Infect. Dis. *13*, 660–662.

LEVINE, M.M. and LEVINE, O.S. 1994. Changes in human ecology and behavior in relation to the emergence of diarrheal diseases, including cholera. Proc. Natl. Acad. Sci. *91*, 2390–2394.

LIPSKY, B.A., HOOK, E.W., SMITH, A.A. and PIORDE, J.J. 1980. Citrobacter infections in humans: experience at the Seattle Veterans Administration Medical Center and a review of the literature. Rev. Infect. Dis. *2*, 746–760.

MESLIN, F.-X. 1997. Global aspects of emerging and potential zoonoses: a WHO perspective. Emerg. Infect. Dis. *3*, 223–228.

MISHU, B. *et al.* 1991. *Salmonella enteritidis* gastroenteritis transmitted by intact chicken eggs. Ann. Intern. Med. *115*, 190–194.

MOOI, F.R. and BIK, E.M. 1997. The evolution of epidemic *Vibrio cholerae* strains. Trends Microbiol. *5*, 161–165.

MOXON, E.R. and MURPHY, P.A. 1978. *Haemophilus influenzae* bacteremia and meningitis resulting from survival of a single organism. Proc. Natl. Acad. Sci. *75*, 1534–1536.

MOXON, E.R., RAINEY, P.B., NOWAK, M.A. and LENSKI, R.E. 1994. Adaptive evolution of highly mutable loci in pathogenic bacteria. Curr. Biol. *4*, 24–33.

MUSMANNO, R.A., RUSSI, M., LIOR, H. and FIGURA, N. 1997. *In vitro* virulence factors of *Arcobacter butzleri* strains isolated from superficial water samples. Microbiologica *20*, 63–68.

NATHANSON, N. 1997. The emergence of infectious diseases: societal causes and consequences. ASM News *63*, 83–88.

ON, S.L.W., STACEY, A. and SMYTH, J. 1995. Isolation of *Arcobacter butzleri* from a neonate with bacteraemia. J. Infect. *31*, 225–227.

PUPO, G.M., KARAOLIS, D.K., LAND, R. and REEVES, P.R. 1997. Evolutionary relationships among pathogenic and nonpathogenic *Escherichia coli* strains inferred from multilocus enzyme electrophoresis and *mdh* sequence studies. Infect. Immun. *65*, 2685–2692.

RASMUSSEN, M.A., CRAY, W.C., CASEY, T.A. and WHIPP, S.C. 1993. Rumen contents as a reservoir of enterohemorrhagic *Escherichia coli*. FEMS Microbiol. Lett. *114*, 79–84.

RAYMOND, G.J. *et al.* 1997. Molecular assessment of the potential transmissibilities of BSE and scrapie to humans. Nature *388*, 285–288.

SAMONIS, G., ANAISSIE, E., ELTING, L. and BODEY, G.P. 1991. Review of *Citrobacter* bacteremia in cancer patients over sixteen-year period. Eur. J. Clin. Microbiol. Infect. Dis. *10*, 479–485.

SCHMIDT, H. *et al.* 1993. Shiga-like toxin II-related cytotoxins in *Citrobacter freundii* strains from humans and beef samples. Infect. Immun. *61*, 534–543.

SCHUCHAT, A., SWAMINATHAN, B. and BROOME, C.V. 1991. Epidemiology of human listeriosis. Clin. Microbiol. Rev. *4*, 169–183.

SHARMA, C. *et al.* 1997. Molecular characterization of *Vibrio cholerae* O1 El Tor Strains isolated between 1992 and 1995 in Calcutta, India: evidence for the emergence of a new clone of the El Tor biotype. J. Infect. Dis. *175*, 1134–1141.

SMITH, J.L. and FRATAMICO, P.M. 1995. Factors involved in the emergence and persistence of food-borne diseases. J. Food Prot. *58*, 696–708.

ST. LOUIS, M.E. *et al.* 1988. The emergence of grade A eggs as a major source of *Salmonella enteritidis* infections. New implications for the control of salmonellosis. J. Am. Med. Assoc. *259*, 2103–2107.

STANLEY, J., GOLDSWORTHY, M. and TRELFALL, E.J. 1992. Molecular phylogenetic typing of pandemic isolates of *Salmonella enteritidis*. FEMS MIcrobiol. Lett. *90*, 153–160.

STILES, M.E. 1989. Less recognized or presumptive foodborne pathogenic bacteria, p. 673–733. In *Foodborne Bacterial Pathogens*, (M.P. Doyle, ed.), Marcel Dekker, New York.

SWERDLOW, D.L. *et al.* 1992. Waterborne transmission of epidemic cholera in Trujillo, Peru: lessons for a continent at risk. Lancet *340*, 28–32.

TAPPERO, J.W., SCHUCHAT, A., DEAVER, K.A., MASCOLA, L. and WENGER, J.D. 1995. Reduction in the incidence of human listeriosis in the United States. J. Am. Med. Assoc. *273*, 118–112.

TILDEN, J. *et al.* 1996. A new route of transmission for *Escherichia coli*: infection from dry fermented salami. Am. J. Pub. Health *86*, 1142–1145.

TSCHÄPE, H. *et al.* 1995. Verotoxigenic *Citrobacter freundii* associated with severe gastroenteritis and cases of haemolytic uraemic syndrome in a nursery school: green butter as the infection source. Epidemiol. Infect. *114S*, 441–450.

WALLACE, J.S., CHEASTY, T. and JONES, K. 1997. Isolation of vero cytotoxin-producing *Escherichia coli* O157 from wild birds. J. Appl. Microbiol. *82*, 399–404.

WATERMAN, S.R. and SMALL, P.L.C. 1996. Characterization of the acid resistance phenotype and *rpoS* alleles of Shiga-like toxin-producing *Escherichia coli*. Infect. Immun. *64*, 2808–3811.

WHITTAM, T. S., WACHSMUTH, I.K. and WILSON, R.A. 1988. Genetic evidence of clonal descent of *Escherichia coli* O157:H7 associated with hemorrhagic colitis and hemolytic uremic syndrome. J. Infect. Dis. *157*, 1124–1133.

WHITTAM, T.S. and WILSON, R.A. 1988. Genetic relationship among pathogenic *Escherichia coli* of serogroup O157. Infect. Immun. 2467–2473.

WHITTAM, T.S. *et al.* 1993. Clonal relationships among *Escherichia coli* strains that cause hemorrhagic colitis and infantile diarrhea. Infect. Immun. *61*, 1619–1629.

WILL, R.G. *et al.* 1996. A new variant of Creutzfeldt-Jakob disease in the UK. Lancet *347*, 921–925.

ZANETTI, F., VAROLI, O., STAMPI, S. and de LUCA, G. 1996. Prevalence of thermophilic *Campylobacter* and *Arcobacter butzleri* in food or animal origin. Internat. J. Food Microbiol. *33*, 315–321.

CHAPTER 8

TWENTY FIVE YEARS OF GENETIC ENGINEERING: A RECORD OF SAFETY AND ACHIEVEMENT

DAVID McCONNELL

Department of Genetics
Trinity College
Dublin, Ireland

ABSTRACT

Genetic engineering developed rapidly following some key discoveries which were made in the 1970s. It has become a set of standard research tools to the extent that it is now commonplace; it is used in many fields of biology, medicine and agriculture by tens of thousands of research scientists world-wide. A quarter of a century of experience shows that while genetic engineering has conceivable risks attached to it there are no substantiated reports of harmful effects, and certainly none of any magnitude. On the contrary, genetic engineering is widely regarded as one of the single most powerful research technologies available. It has been one of the main reasons for a revolution in knowledge of biological systems and for many novel beneficial products and processes affecting daily life. The best known example is human insulin. Cheeses, beers and other foods and drinks are produced more efficiently and to the same, if not higher, standards because of genetic engineering. This paper considers the general theory and technology of genetic engineering, its regulation, the public perception of risks, the safety record, some applications to food production and processing, some accusations that genetic engineering of food has caused harm, some benefits which have accrued and the prospects for the future. The paper concludes that genetically modified foods are likely to be as good for us as traditional foods. Genetic engineering is adding value to food at minimal risk; in some cases it will reduce risks and it may increase world food production. Unlike many other technologies, genetic engineering has had a twenty five year harm-free record, a good omen for the future but not a guarantee.

INTRODUCTION

There has been much public, professional and political concern about genetic engineering since the emergence of the technology in the 1970s. Recently, in

Europe some of this concern has been concentrated on the safety of genetically engineered food and has been well-reported in the media. The general anxiety about food safety is well-justified by the emergence of the prion causing BSE, as well as *Listeria* and *E. coli* O157:H7, which are serious threats to humans and farm animals. People are now more aware than ever of the general danger of food-poisoning, but the concerns have some of the qualities of hysteria in that some of the risks are not as high as perceived, some real risks are being ignored, and innocent parties are shouldering some of the blame. Geneticists in particular have been caught in this tidal wave of public concern about food. It is proposed here that the concerns about genetics are almost completely without foundation.

Part of the concern about genetically engineered food arises from alarmist reactions to the use of genetic engineering in medicine and related fields. Many people believe wrongly that genetic engineering is inherently dangerous. In fact genetic engineering is contributing enormously to modern medicine and has an impeccable safety record. According to James Watson, Nobel prizewinner:

"To my knowledge ... not one case of recombinant DNA-induced illness has ... occurred. No person has been killed, nor has even one case of serious illness been attributed to recombinant DNA, nor do we know of any case where the release into nature of any recombinant DNA-modified organism has led to any known ecological disaster. This is not to say that someday a recombinant DNA-induced disease will not occur. Today, however, there is certainly no logical reason for not exploiting recombinant DNA procedures as fast as possible for human betterment" (Watson 1996).

The concerns about the effects of genetics on food are probably diverting attention from other more substantial dangers which arise from the natural biology of food, for example (1) the threat of pathogenic microbial contamination arising during production, processing, transport, storage, display or preparation of food, and (2) the misuse or overuse of artificial chemicals in agriculture or processing.

Applied genetics is regulated according to laws which vary little between countries in the Organisation for Economic Cooperation and Development (OECD) and poses no significant threat to the safety of food. It is a constructive and beneficial science which has contributed substantially to the health and welfare of all peoples; it should be supported as important for the food security of the world in the next century. It should of course be regulated but the regulations should reflect the magnitude of real and not imaginary risks.

The subject is addressed in three sections devoted to pre-scientific genetics, classical genetics and genetic engineering. The record of pre-scientific genetics (8,000 BC to 1900 AD) and of classical genetics (1900 - present) is clear — the world population could not have increased to its current level without the discoveries and developments made through *the completely safe application* of pre-scientific and classical genetics which underlie the whole of agriculture. The third phase of agricultural genetics is now being unfolded, through the application of plant and animal genetic engineering (1970 - present).

There is no reason to expect a different verdict when the history of this third phase of genetics comes to be written — there is already 25 years of safe experience of genetic engineering on which to base this prediction and there are few, if any, risks which can be foreseen on reasonable grounds. Of course mistakes, or even disasters, cannot be ruled out but the record so far is perfect and the understanding of the biology is sound. Geneticists have not been and are not irresponsible. Even if disasters are unlikely, vigilance is required especially by the professional scientists and the professional regulators who are in the best position to notice problems. The prospective benefits, however, far outweigh the risks which can be reasonably identified at the present time. At the risk of leaving hostages to fortune, it seems likely that genetic engineering will not cause many, if any problems, which are qualitatively different from those already known within the general practice of agriculture.

PRE-SCIENTIFIC GENETICS (8,000 BC TO 1900 AD)

Pre-scientific genetics was, in the first instance, responsible for the transition from hunter-gatherer to farming societies. The story of the discovery of agriculture has been told by Diamond (1997) and Smith (1995). The first farmers seem to have appeared in the Fertile Crescent about 10,000 years ago. Their society was based on the domestication of the genes of what Diamond has called the eight "founder crops" - emmer wheat, einkorn wheat, barley, pea, chickpea, lentil, bitter vetch and flax. Farming actually developed independently in several parts of the world, always piecemeal and sometimes very slowly, with the domestication of appropriate sets of local species, for example rice and two millets in China, sorghum and pearl millet in Africa, sugar cane in New Guinea and corn (maize) in the Americas. The dog (wolf) was the first relatively large mammal to be domesticated, probably first in China about 10,000 years ago. Cow, pig, goat and sheep were domesticated about 6 to 8,000 years ago in the Fertile Crescent, and the horse in the Ukraine about 4,000 years ago.

The overall result is that a relatively small number of plants and animals have been domesticated by man, a tiny fraction of the number of available species. There are several hundred thousand species of plants; a few thousand are eaten by man and a few hundred have been domesticated for food production. This choice of species is itself an example of pre-scientific genetic selection; plants and animals were chosen which were known from experience to be palatable and nutritious, which gave reliable high natural yields, which in some cases could be stored and had other valuable qualities. For the animals a key property was whether they could be domesticated.

From these early times only a few thousand years ago until the present day, *Homo sapiens* has been applying genetics to the production of "better" foods. The basic pre-scientific genetic technique is simple and is well-known to all: choose (select) and breed from the parental stock which has the most advantageous characteristics. If this is done, these characteristics will improve generation after generation. Hybridisation between different species followed by selection of successful progeny, which often occurs to a limited extent in the wild and can therefore be said to be "natural", was also practiced. Whether unwittingly or not is immaterial, hybridisation gave rise thousands of years ago to several of the most important modern crops, for example, modern wheat.

There are many primitive examples of the specificity of pre-scientific selection by ancient man. Wild almonds are bitter due to amygdalin which breaks down to produce enough cyanide per almond for a few to kill a person. Man discovered and propagated rare mutant trees which did not produce amygdalin. Other plants whose wild parents produce toxins which have been selected out in the process of domestication include lima beans, cabbage, potatoes, eggplants and watermelons (Diamond 1997).

CLASSICAL GENETICS (1900 AD TO THE PRESENT)

The word *bios*, Greek for life, was not applied in the scientific sense which is now common (anything to do with life in the broadest sense, biology, biosphere, etc.) until the 19th century. Until then *bios* meant life, a supernatural quality possessed by man and only by man. In the 19th century, biology emerged as the scientific study of living things. As the Concise Oxford English Dictionary says in a somewhat dated way, the prefix "bio-" has been "extended ... in modern formations ... to include organic life" (Anon. 1950). Now the prefix "bio-" is being used in a way which has completely obscured the pre-19th century origin and usage.

The dictionary entry is a tiny reflection of the 19th century revolution in biology. This was stimulated by some remarkable scientists who are household names, e.g. Bernard, the founder of physiology and biochemistry and Mendel, the father of genetics. Interestingly, in view of the subject of this paper, it is possible that the 19th century revolution in biology owed a great deal to an on-going revolution in farming. The industrial revolution and the concomitant population explosion and growth of cities, led to huge demands for food. Farming began to industrialise. Pressures intensified for higher yielding plants and animals. New varieties, such as sugar beet, appeared in the 18th century derived from beet varieties grown "since Babylonian times" for their edible roots and leaves.

The impact of agriculture is easily seen. Darwin and Mendel were greatly influenced by observations on farming and horticulture, especially on the species which had been domesticated and the massive amount of heritable variation which could be seen when different breeds of the same species were compared. Darwin's description of the effects of artificial selection on domestic plants and animals, for example on domestic pigeons by pigeon fanciers, forms an important part of his argument for natural selection. Darwin placed natural variation (with natural selection) as one of the two principles at the centre of his theory of evolution. Mendel, an Augustinian monk in the monastery of Brno, was carrying on the tradition of agriculture and horticulture so important to monastic life since the early middle ages. He knew about the ways in which local farmers propagated seed from year to year to ensure good crops, and especially about the variation between varieties in garden peas. Before he became Abbott he was in charge of the monastery garden. Within a few years the two greatest discoveries in biology were described by men who were knowledgeable gardeners. Darwin's "On The Origin of Species" was published in 1859; Mendel's paper on the mechanism of inheritance in garden peas which identified inherited factors which are now called genes, was published in 1866.

Mendel's work was rediscovered in 1900 and the new science of genetics quickly emerged. The re-birth and development of genetics was closely followed by plant and animal breeders and the new science began to provide a powerful theoretical framework for plant and animal breeding; the rate of improvement of plant varieties and animal breeds accelerated. By 1950 all the major domesticated crops and animal breeds used for food production in the western world were being subjected to massive scientific breeding programmes, sometimes organised by seed companies, sometimes by growers and sometimes by governments. In Ireland, major breeding programmes were carried out by the Irish Sugar Company on sugar beet, by the Department of Agriculture and Food on wheat and by the malsters on malting barley. The Irish co-operatives began to use genetics in selecting pedigree bulls for AI services. Before any bull went into wide service it was subjected to one round of "progeny testing" and compared with its "competitors". The animals with the best genetic merit went into service and the remainder were sold or culled. This process has led to substantial increases in milk and meat production.

The production of all foods from domesticated species has grown steadily in the 20th century in Europe, the Americas and Australasia, partly through the use of the more productive varieties and breeds which were the outcome of massive genetic breeding programmes, and partly through other modern agronomic innovations (fertilisers, etc). But the developing world lagged behind, suffering frequently from famines. The developing world awaited the application of classical genetics and modern methods of plant and animal husbandry.

The Green Revolution is a term used to describe the extraordinary increase in world food production which began in the developing world about 1950 and is still under way. In the 1950s and even in the 1960s famine was a major threat in Asia, notably in India and China. Food production lagged behind the population boom, more or less the way it had in Europe in the 19th century, when famine was also widespread. The Rockefeller and Ford Foundations began to invest in plant breeding programmes for rice and wheat, the most important Asian crops, and very important in most of the developing world. They supported the foundation of two institutes, a wheat breeding institute in Mexico and a rice breeding institute in the Philippines. The International Rice Research Institute (IRRI) was opened at Los Banos, in the Philippines in 1960. The Institute is sponsored by the United Nations, FAO, the World Bank and the United Nations Development Programme (UNDP). It is one of 13 Consultative Groups on International Agricultural Research (CGIAR) non-profit international research and training centres to which about 50 countries, as well as private donors and foundations, make financial contributions. The impact has been remarkable even measured in terms of education — 5000 rice scientists have been trained since 1986.

More importantly, IRRI began to collect and store seed from species and land races (varieties) of rice from throughout the world, and to use these to breed higher yielding hybrid rice. By 1986 IRRI had collected more than 75,000 of the estimated 120,000 extant varieties. These were cultivated and classified as to yield, resistance to fungi and other pathogens, tendency to lodge, susceptibility to drought, response to fertilisers and so forth. Of course no single variety was top for all qualities. Through hybridisation and selection new varieties which combined important qualities were developed. The scale of the enterprise is impressive. About 4000 crosses are made per year with the progeny distributed for testing in various habitats.

Years of painstaking research led to the development of a series of varieties which gave very high yields and were resistant to pests. In 1966 the strain IR8 was released for general use; it was essentially a cross between a semi-dwarf short-stemmed Chinese strain which allowed the plants to respond to high levels of fertiliser without lodging, and a tall vigorous Indonesian strain. Yields were doubled or tripled. In 1985 the strain IR64 was released with better grain quality, disease resistance and lodging resistance. It out-yielded its predecessor IR36 by about 20% in 16 experimental stations over 4 seasons. IR64 had genes from 20 original land races from 8 countries. The new strains have been distributed around the world. India has not had a famine for decades and China is now a net exporter of rice. Rice yields per country increased by about 2 fold from 1950 to 1980.

In summary, classical genetics has provided a theoretical basis for a large increase in the genetic merit of many important domesticated species of plants and animals from 1900 to the present day. It has been estimated that the productivity of the major species which have been worked on (wheat, rice, cattle, corn, etc.) has been increasing by 1% per annum due to genetics. Much more can be achieved, especially through the application of classical genetics to other crops and animals, especially to those from arid and semi-arid climates, and in the animal world to fish and shellfish.

GENETIC ENGINEERING

In the broad sense all plant and animal breeding is genetic engineering. Until about 1980 almost all genetic engineering in food and agriculture was based on the theories and knowledge of classical genetics. In the narrow sense and by common usage, the term genetic engineering is applied to those experimental manipulations involving recombinant DNA, a technology which was invented about 1970 and which began to be applied to food production, at first indirectly, from about 1980. The narrow definition is merely a technical definition telling us about how we might change the genetics of an organism using a certain DNA-based technology. Man has been engineering change in the genetics of organisms for about 10,000 years; in other words genetic engineering in the broad sense has been ongoing for a very long time.

There is a clear and continuous connection between broad sense genetic engineering and narrow sense genetic engineering — one technology led directly to the other and they are carried out by members of the same profession. Importantly the narrow sense technology cannot be applied usefully to plants and animals without using broad-sense genetic engineering technology, i.e, the classical methods of plant and animal breeding. It is important to emphasise the continuity of applied genetics; there are no new hidden agendas and no new principles. Geneticists have not suddenly changed their professional objectives and are still motivated largely by the desire to increase human knowledge and human welfare.

Genetic engineering, defined in the narrow sense except where indicated, is a technology which allows the isolation of any gene from any organism and its transfer to any other organism, even to a member of a different species in such a way that the gene will operate in the recipient organism and be passed on to its offspring.

Genes are made of DNA, a chemical which is present in all cells of all organisms. It can be extracted from cells and purified as a colourless substance, soluble in water and quite stable. It is a long and thin chemical, which has some of the qualities of a tape for a tape recorder. In other words a gene is a long stretch of linear information which can be read out or remain dormant. A gene can be compared to a song on a long tape with many songs. Just like a song on a tape, a gene has a beginning and an end. Between the beginning and the end there is information which, in the case of a gene, causes a protein to be made. So a golden rule of molecular genetics is that one gene codes for one protein. Proteins are made of a different chemical substance than DNA; they are the key sub-cellular work-horses of organisms. Examples include haemoglobin (made of two proteins α and β globin) which carries oxygen in blood cells, rhodopsin which is the light-receptor in the rod cells of the retina, immunoglobulins which are antibodies, enzymes, insulin and growth hormone. Man (and other mammals) has between 100,000 and 1,000,000 genes, coding therefore for the same number of proteins. Higher plants have about the same number of genes as man.

DNA is a polymer, a linear array of four different kinds of chemical sub-units called for short A, C, T and G. The sequence of these sub-units (A, C, T and G are collectively called bases) is the genetic information. Different genes have different sequences of A, C, T and G. A simple gene has an average of 1000 bases. There is a code which relates the base sequence to the structure of the corresponding protein and this code is essentially universal, i.e., it has the same relationship in all organisms.

To continue the analogy with a recording tape it is of course possible to copy or replicate a tape. DNA can also be replicated. Each cell has a complete set of genes and these have to be replicated just before a cell divides. And genes have to be controlled so that the appropriate proteins are produced in each cell type. The globins are only made in red blood cells, strictly in the precursor cell type which is called a reticulocyte, and this implies that the globin genes must be turned off in all other cell types. This is achieved by information stored in the DNA between the genes. Between songs on a tape there is usually a stretch which is silent. Between genes in a DNA molecule there is a stretch which is not quite silent — it contains the code which controls the gene next to it.

Avery *et al.* (1944) at Rockefeller University in New York provided the first evidence that genes were made of DNA and the structure of DNA was discovered by Watson and Crick (1953). By 1961 the mechanism by which DNA coded for protein, by which protein production was regulated, by which DNA replicated and by which it mutated (the basic process of Darwinian evolution) had been deduced. Mutations are changes in the base sequence of the DNA, one base change being sufficient to make a very significant, even lethal, change.

Smith (1970), working at Johns Hopkins University in Baltimore, discovered a kind of enzyme called a type II restriction enzyme, which chops DNA in a specific manner into lengths which are about gene-sized. If the DNA molecule was short, for example the DNA molecule from a virus, it was quite easy to separate the fragments of DNA from each other and so purify individual genes.

Different American laboratories discovered an enzyme, DNA ligase, which could join DNA molecules together (Little *et al.* 1967). It was possible to use this enzyme to join not just the same but different DNA molecules. In other words it was possible to create new combinations of DNA molecules, that is to produce recombinant DNA. DNA molecules from different organisms could be joined together. Recombinant DNA molecules were first made from bacterial and viral DNA in California at Stanford University and at the University of California at San Francisco (Cohen *et al.* 1973). The recombinant DNA molecules were re-introduced into bacteria and shown to function. This procedure is called molecular cloning, which must be distinguished from the cloning of organisms. These experiments opened up ways for the purification of any gene and the transfer of genes from one species to another.

It took only a short time for people to realise that this technology could be useful. American and European university scientists set up the first biotechnology companies, notably Genentech in California and Biogen in Massachusetts and Europe in 1975-76 and the race was on to produce the first valuable pharmaceutical. One important target was human insulin for diabetics who were then being treated with pig insulin. The human insulin gene was isolated and put into the bacterium *E. coli* (or, by another laboratory, into baker's yeast) and the microbes were thus re-programmed to make insulin. Today almost all diabetics are treated with human insulin made by genetically engineered microbes. Biogen, developed the first genetically engineered human vaccine, one which gives protection against hepatitis B. This vaccine is used by most people travelling to tropical and sub-tropical countries where hepatitis B is endemic and a major cause of both hepatitis and liver cancer. Other major genetically engineered pharmaceutical products include the interferons and interleukins used against cancer, growth hormone to treat genetic dwarfs, enzymes as therapy for children with certain inborn errors of metabolism such as Gaucher's Disease and erythropoietin used to stimulate blood production, for example in patients after kidney transplantation.

The pharmaceutical industry is being revolutionised by the technology of genetic engineering. Companies are sequencing the complete genetic code of pathogenic viruses and bacteria to decode the genetic information which makes them pathogenic. The principle behind this approach is the equivalent of espionage. The DNA of a pathogen, the enemy, has the plan for attacking the defender. If the plan can be seen and deciphered it should be possible to wreck the attacker or to plan a good defence. The best example of this strategy is the analysis of HIV which causes AIDS. The virus was discovered and defined using genetic engineering technology. The base sequence of the virus immediately suggested how specific new drugs might be designed to combat AIDS. The new triple therapy includes one such drug. Other examples under study by genetic engineering are the bacterium *Helicobacter pylori* which causes ulcers and cancer, *Mycobacterium tubercle* which causes tuberculosis, and *Mycobacterium leprae* which causes leprosy. The DNA sequence of these bacteria may well reveal new methods for therapy (defense) and new antibiotics (attack).

Even more remarkable, there is a huge, loosely co-ordinated, international consortium of geneticists which is sequencing human DNA, believing that this will help to explain why humans are susceptible to many different kinds of disease, especially cancers, genetic diseases and diseases of old age. This project will be completed by about the year 2005.

In summary, genetic engineering is a set of experimental procedures which have been applied routinely in biology laboratories for a quarter of a century. Many important fundamental discoveries have been made which have revolutionised different fields of biology: ribozymes, enzymes made of RNA and thought now to have been important at an early stage in prebiotic evolution; the mechanism for the generation of diversity of immunoglobulins; the discovery that BSE and other similar diseases, including kuru and scrapie are caused by prions, infectious agents which do not contain DNA and seem to act as molecular chaperones; the genetic basis of inherited blindness; the genetic basis of cancer, including certain forms of breast cancer; the discovery that some people are genetically prone to having children with spina bifida; verification of Kimura's neutral theory of molecular evolution; substantiation and calibration of the molecular clock; proof that all humans are descended from a small group of people who probably lived in Africa 150,000 years ago; evidence that Neanderthal Man belonged to a different species than *Homo sapiens* and has left no descendants, etc. The avalanche of knowledge and the rapidly evolving methods of experimentation and analysis are being applied to problems in medicine, agriculture and industry and they are impacting on such diverse fields as philosophy, ethics and forensics. It is reasonable to suggest that genetic engineering has revolutionised human knowledge and advanced human welfare to a significant extent.

Examples of detrimental effects of genetic engineering in the past 25 years are unknown. Claims that it has caused damage or even death cannot be substantiated. There is a claim that a strain of bacteria which was used to produce tryptophan, a food additive, caused a number of deaths *because* the strain was genetically engineered. This does not appear to be true. The strain was indeed genetically engineered and deaths did occur, but the poison has been identified and traced to a change in the process of purifying the tryptophan.

Tens of thousands of genetic engineering experiments are in progress every day in laboratories all over the world. They vary in sophistication from simple experiments, which can be done in a school laboratory, to hugely complex experiments which need large teams of skilled scientists and expensive high technology laboratories and equipment.

GENETIC ENGINEERING AND FOOD

It is important to realise that there are two general ways in which genetic engineering is affecting the production of food; first through the genetic engineering of food plants and animals themselves, and second through the provision of enzymes (and other substances) which are used in food processing.

The first example relates to cheese and a well known step in cheese production, the production of the curd. Traditionally this was carried out by adding an extract of calf stomach (called rennet) to the milk. The rennet contains an enzyme called rennin which chemically attacks the milk protein called casein causing the milk to clot. The clotted curd can then be separated from the whey and the cheese formed and allowed to mature. By 1970 a shortage of calf stomachs was becoming apparent (because it was more valuable to allow the calves to grow into adult animals). Scientists discovered that other enzymes could be used as substitutes for rennin, some from fungi for example, but they were not satisfactory for all cheeses. The solution to this problem was to take the gene for rennin from cow DNA and put it into bacteria, which would then be programmed to make as much rennin as necessary. Apart from rescuing the international cheese industry, this would allow some vegetarians to eat cheese.

This rennin was introduced internationally on the basis that there were no conceivable dangers due to the genetic engineering and that good manufacturing practice (hygienic production, non-pathogenic organism as the production strain, insignificant microbial contamination of the product, etc.) would ensure that the product carried no dangers. In theory and practice making cheese with genetically engineered rennin is an entirely safe process.

The second example, enzymes, concerns the food and drink industry in a more general way. Many foods are processed by the use of enzymes which break down high molecular weight materials such as proteins, fats and carbohydrates. For example, in making bread some of the starch in the flour is broken into smaller pieces by enzymes which are produced by the baker's yeast. This gives the bread its texture and makes it digestible by the less effective enzymes in the stomach. When meat ages, enzymes in the meat begin to degrade the meat. Fruits ripen through the activity of enzymes. Enzymatic digestion is a normal part of the "natural" processes of baking, brewing, wine-making, pickling, salting, tea and coffee production, cheese-making, yoghurt-making, etc. Of course, once food is taken in it is digested with enzymes first in the mouth and then in the stomach and blood stream.

Food processing can be made more efficient by the addition of enzymes. If jam is made at home, pectin, a kind of sugary polymer, can be added to help to set the jam. But pectin, which comes from the skins of fruits, has an unhappy but perfectly harmless effect of making fruit juice cloudy. So fruit-juice makers may add an enzyme called pectinase to digest the pectin and prevent cloudiness.

Such food processing enzymes are often produced today by genetically-engineered bacteria or yeasts. They are used in such a large number of different foods and drinks that it is probably impossible to avoid eating some processed food or drink in a normal diet which has not involved the use of a genetically engineered product in the processing. In terms of safety these enzymes are produced under rigorous conditions with standards comparable to those in the pharmaceutical industry and they pose no special hazards which have been introduced because of the application of genetic engineering.

Finally to genetically engineered plants. Monsanto and its associated companies have produced a series of varieties of sugar beet which are resistant to a herbicide called *Roundup*. This herbicide is available in all garden centres. The evidence shows that it is essentially safe, that it does not persist in soil and does not produce harmful residues. The sugar beet varieties produced by pre-scientific and classical genetic engineering from the 18th century onwards are sensitive to *Roundup*. Monsanto have used genetic engineering (recombinant DNA) to make sugar beet varieties resistant to *Roundup* by adding a gene for *Roundup* resistance. *Roundup* can therefore be used to spray fields sown with these varieties; it is claimed that this will give higher yields to the farmer. There has been considerable objection to using these varieties in Europe even though the project has been examined by different geneticists and agronomists and has passed many official investigations in the United States and elsewhere, and found to be safe. It appears that these sugar beet varieties are without any conceivable danger and public opposition is misdirected.

A second example is related to an experiment with a bacterial protein called BT which kills certain insects. The BT toxin has been widely used as a "biological insecticide" for many years. BT producing bacteria can be grown in large quantities and simply sprayed onto crops; BT is close to the ultimate in "green" technology.

A bacterial gene for the BT toxin has been transferred into plants. These plants are resistant to caterpillars. This kind of experiment has far reaching implications for all plants which are destroyed by insect larvae. Essentially the plants have acquired a single new gene which allows each plant to produce its own insecticidal toxin. The only insects which are killed are those which eat the plant, which is a much more specific procedure than spraying.

Genetic engineering projects of this general kind are under way in the United States and Europe to produce more valuable plants and there are a few experiments under way to genetically engineer animals. Long-lasting tomatoes have been made and are on sale. Plants can in principle be made which produce human proteins, for example human insulin, and they might be more efficient than the bacteria or yeast which are used at the moment. In Edinburgh, Dolly the sheep has been made, opening the long-term objective of breeding sheep or other animals which could make human proteins (Wilmut 1997).

It is worthwhile comparing the precision of the method of genetic engineering by recombinant DNA with the pre-scientific and classical methods of genetic engineering which have been used so successfully for 10,000 years and 100 years, respectively. The older methods were very much hit and miss, with hybridisations involving the mixing of millions of genes and with no chance of complete control of the outcome of an "experiment". In contrast, modern genetic engineering has the precision of changing one or a very few genes at a time and in a pre-determined way with exquisite molecular finesse.

RISKS ASSOCIATED WITH GENETIC ENGINEERING OF FOOD AND FOOD INGREDIENTS

Although the record of genetic engineering so far has been perfect, a number of risks to food, agriculture and ecosystems have been considered, mostly associated with genetically engineered plants.

It has been suggested that the single genes introduced into domesticated plants might "escape" into related wild plants or even into related domestic plants and that this would be dangerous or deleterious. There is no doubt that some such "escapes" will occur and indeed such transfers have been documented in experimental plots. Such escapes pose no special danger which can be said to be specifically associated with the fact that the donor plants have been genetically engineered. This means that genes may conceivably "escape" from any plant to close relatives and less likely to more distantly-related species; this is not something which arises specifically in the case of genetically engineered plants or animals.

The escape of an individual gene from a genetically engineered plant will have no effect on the genetic make-up of the recipient plants as a species unless it spreads through the recipient population. According to the basic principles of population genetics it can only spread by two methods. Either it provides a selective advantage or it spreads (through a small population) by genetic drift. For example, *Roundup* which would be the selection pressure of the gene for *Roundup* resistance, will not usually be applied outside the fields. So the gene will not spread outside the fields. One can imagine that the gene might build up in weeds, through transfer from the crop and subsequent selection within plots of land which are consistently treated with *Roundup*. Otherwise a gene may spread by drift but only if the recipient population is very small and thus insignificant.

It may be argued that it would not be good for agriculture if a *Roundup* resistance gene were to spread from a resistant crop into weeds which are at present controlled by *Roundup*. In the first instance this is unlikely because weeds are usually not closely related to crops. Secondly this kind of matter is very carefully considered by the manufacturers and the regulatory authorities. The manufacturers will not want to create a situation which neutralises the value of their product and the regulatory agency will not authorise the release of a genetically engineered crop which is likely to neutralise a very important weedkiller. It cannot be guaranteed that this will never happen, but the likelihood can be judged. Genetically engineered crops are only approved when such transfers are judged to be very unlikely. If it does happen by hybridisation that a closely related and important weed becomes resistant to a valuable herbicide then so be it — that herbicide will not be as useful and in the extreme case the weedkiller will no longer be useful at all.

The use of *Roundup* may in principle also select for rare natural resistance mutants in weed populations. However *Roundup* resistance is apparently very rare, with no case of a spontaneous resistant weed appearing since *Roundup* was introduced more than 20 years ago. But if this occurs it will be a price that may have to be paid for the use of this herbicide in the same way as a price is being paid for the use of certain antibiotics. However, no one ever suggests that antibiotics should not have been discovered or used. Their use should have been better controlled and of course the use of herbicides should be carefully controlled. Proper regulation of the use of herbicides should take into account the fact that many more crops are going to be engineered to become herbicide resistant but there is no need to limit arbitrarily the practice of genetic engineering. In some cases genetic engineering may well lead to a reduction in the use herbicides because different treatment regimes may be possible and also to the use of herbicides which are preferable as less expensive, less toxic and less likely to lead to naturally occurring resistant mutants.

Of course, natural populations need to be protected from genetic introgression. Consider the case of the Simian jackal of Ethiopia *Canis simensis* which is threatened with extinction because it is hybridising with domestic dogs, but such problems will hardly ever have anything to do with genetic engineering and are not likely to be exacerbated by genetic engineering.

A second risk which has been suggested is that genetic engineering will lead to a reduction in biodiversity, which is difficult to understand. It is true that some practices in agriculture, horticulture and forestry lead to vast monocultures, say of sitka spruce in Ireland, or maize in North America. Agriculture has destroyed or irrevocably altered great tracts of the natural environment, but these processes are not going to be altered by genetic engineering. The destruction of the natural environment is regretted but, apart from minor adjustments, the clock cannot be turned back in the immediate future. Things will get a lot worse in Africa, Asia and South America, and indeed on many small islands, until the population stabilises. More efficient food production will also help and genetic engineering will be important in increasing food production per hectare.

On the plus side for genetics, a great deal of effort has been put into discovering or developing and preserving rare breeds of animals or plants during the last 10,000 years. The most obvious example is the domestic dog. All dogs are domesticated wolves and over thousands of years man has selectively bred from those rare animals which had attractive or useful characteristics which would have been lost if not chosen and protected by man. Less obviously note should be taken of the large number of breeds of domestic cattle, many hundreds of distinguishable breeds selected by man for their special qualities useful in a great range of different environments. Today special efforts are being made to conserve rare breeds precisely because geneticists have been emphasising their value in enriching the gene pool. The huge library of rice species has already been mentioned and land races assembled by IRRI at Los Banos in the Philippines. It was Bateson the great British geneticist of the early 1900s who said "Treasure your exceptions" an injunction followed to this day by all geneticists because genetic diversity is the stuff of their science.

A third criticism concerns the possibility that genetically engineered herbicide-resistant plants may themselves become weeds, uncontrollable by the herbicide in question. This possibility is examined on a case by case basis by the regulatory authorities even though it is extremely unlikely simply because domesticated plants are usually unable to compete in the wild. Introduced plants (prickly pear in Australia, sycamore and Buddleia in Ireland and European gorse in New Zealand) are examples of the very large number of introduced wild plants spreading in new territories, so care is needed. But this is not a new problem brought about by genetic engineering and it will not be changed very much by genetic engineering, if at all.

A fourth criticism of genetic engineers is that they are aiding and abetting the genetic plunder of developing countries. They are said to be stealing rare organisms or genes from developing countries and using these third world genes to genetically engineer crops or to produce valuable pharmaceuticals. The novel crops or pharmaceuticals developed in the OECD countries may then be sold to the developing countries who will have to pay for the use of their own genes or gene products. This is a convoluted argument related to the worrying North-South division. In spite of the apparent justice of the argument the case does not stand up to analysis.

The fact is that agricultural and pharmaceutical science, indeed all science, is international. There is no tradition or legal substance to the idea that a country may own an agricultural organism. Countries have tried (Brazil and rubber, perhaps China and tea) but the impracticality of the aspirations has only emphasised the lack of balance of the claims. Even pre-historic science was international in the sense that agriculture was invented in a few places and shared with neighbours and ultimately with the rest of the world. Potatoes from Peru and tomatoes from Mexico are grown all over the world. Mexicans and Peruvians grow wheat and cattle from the Middle East and many other plants and animals from other continents.

New strains of plants and cattle are being bred in many parts of the world and distributed widely, sometimes *gratis* under aid programmes and sometimes by sale. Sale and economic dominance is of course the reason for third world concerns about the use of third world genes by OECD commerce. But sale in a modified and partly regulated free-market is a mechanism which rewards the seller for the cleverness of discovery and the huge investment in development, proof of value, demonstration of safety as well as marketing and distribution. Regulated commercialisation is the best known mechanism for the encouragement of novel product development and it should be allowed to operate in the application of genetic engineering. If, for example, India wishes to place an embargo on the export of any genetic material from India, as it has apparently done, then it might be worthwhile asking whether India will also place an embargo on the import of foreign genetic material or the products which have been produced through genetics, and will India return the genes which have been sent there over the millennia? Clearly this is a debate about protectionism and has to be seen in a wider context. There are third world genes which could be used for the benefit of the peoples of the world but the benefits can be most rapidly distributed through the application of science and industry which are at present mostly located in the universities and corporations of the OECD countries.

Fifthly, it has been argued that some genetically engineered crops have genes which confer resistance to useful antibiotics and these genes may well spread into bacterial pathogens and neutralise the value of certain antibiotics. This is an understandable fear which is based on a nearly complete misunderstanding of biology. It is true that some genetically engineered crops have such antibiotic-resistance genes. They were transferred to the plant by a kind of genetic hitch-hiking in the process of making the genetically-engineered crop. They are not significant to the farmer and the farmer will not be spraying penicillin or any other antibiotic on his crops.

Such antibiotic-resistance genes are most unlikely ever to transfer to any bacteria because genes rarely cross species boundaries, say from man to elephant. Although there are examples, much less often do they cross boundaries between biological kingdoms, say from plant to microbe. They are even less likely to transfer to a pathogenic bacterium and even less likely to transfer to a pathogen which is dangerous to man or domestic livestock. Such organisms are not found in huge numbers near or in crop plants, they are not known to receive genes from plant chromosomes and there are no selective pressures (the antibiotic) to cause such genes to spread through such bacteria if by some quirk they had been picked up.

In contrast to this imaginary risk of the transfer of antibiotic resistance from plant to bacterial pathogens which infect man, there is a real and large risk that dangerous, untreatable antibiotic-resistant bacteria will be selected by the unwise use of antibiotics in animal husbandry.

CONCLUSION

Genetic engineering has a 25 year record of safety. There is ample evidence that genetic engineering has led to remarkable advances in human knowledge and welfare. The technology has been applied with great care under strict regulation with unprecedented caution. The American inventors of the technology and their colleagues actually called a voluntary embargo on experimentation at the famous Asilomar Conference in June 1974. The embargo lasted for 2 years until regulations were drafted in 1975 under the aegis of the National Institutes of Health of the US Government and published in 1976. They have gradually been relaxed as the authorities gained a greater understanding of the risks involved and realised that the only risks worth considering related to studies on genes from pathogenic organisms, or genes which coded for toxic substances. Genetic engineering in Ireland is regulated by the Environmental Protection Agency according to European and Irish law. In retrospect, the wide range of the regulations was unnecessary. But they remain in force for some kinds of experiments and these are necessary when dangerous pathogens are being used, for example when bacteria or viruses which are pathogenic for plants, animals or humans are being studied. It is important to be able to use genetic engineering to study dangerous organisms and the general rule is to use conditions which are determined by the danger of the object of the study.

Unfortunately instead of instilling public confidence, the regulations have added to the alarm of some people in Ireland. The public does not think "big" government can be trusted at all. In the United States, public opinion has moved on to the next stage of realising that "genetic engineering is good for you" and geneticists are usually on the side of the angels. Modern day genetic engineers are carrying on a tradition of 10,000 years, different only in that they are working with much greater knowledge and much greater precision. In comparison to the real threats to health, for example due to poor hygiene in the food processing industry, the consumer has virtually nothing to fear from genetic engineering. It can be expected that food will be cheaper, last longer, taste better or have some other quality which enhances its place in the world-wide marketplace, and more food will be grown in more extreme climates on poorer soils, because of genetic engineering.

REFERENCES

ANON. 1950. Concise Oxford English Dictionary, Clarendon Press, Oxford.

AVERY, O.T., MacLEOD, C.M. and McCART, M. 1944. J. Exp. Med. *78*, 137.

COHEN, S.N., CHANG, A.C.Y., BOYER, and HELLING, R.B. 1973. Construction of biologically functional bacteria plasmids in vitro. Proc. Nat'l. Acad. Sci. USA *70*, 3240–3244.

DIAMOND, J. 1997. Guns, germs and steel: the gates of human societies. W. W. Norton, New York.

LITTLE, J.W., LEHMAN, I.R. and KAISER, A.D. 1967. J. Biol. Chem. *242*, 72.

SMITH, B.D. 1995. The emergence of agriculture. Scientific American Library, New York.

SMITH, H.O. 1970. Nucleotide sequence specificity of restriction endonucleases. Science *205*, 455–462.

WATSON, J. 1996. President's Report, Cold Spring Harbor Laboratory, Long Island, New York.

WATSON, J.D. and CRICK, F.H.C. 1953. Nature *171*, 737.

WILMUT, I. 1997. Viable offspring derived from foetal and adult mammalian cells. Nature, London.

CHAPTER 9

THE DEVELOPMENT OF A RISK ASSESSMENT MODEL FOR USE IN THE POULTRY INDUSTRY

THOMAS P. OSCAR

United States Department of Agriculture
Agricultural Research Service
Microbial Food Safety Research Unit
1124 Trigg Hall
University of Maryland Eastern Shore
Princess Anne, MD 21853

ABSTRACT

A simulation model that assesses the risk of acquiring salmonellosis from consumption and handling of chicken was created in an Excel™ spreadsheet and was simulated using @Risk™. The model simulated the distribution, preparation, and consumption of 1,000 chickens and was designed to determine the relationship between the level of Salmonella *contamination on chickens at the processing plant exit and the risk of salmonellosis for consumers of the chickens. A scatter plot of the probability of acquiring salmonellosis from consumption of the chickens simulated versus the* Salmonella *load on the chickens at the processing plant exit clearly showed that highly (i.e., > 100* Salmonella*/bird) contaminated chickens at the plant exit did not necessarily pose greater risk of salmonellosis than lightly (i.e., < 10* Salmonella*/bird) contaminated chickens at the plant exit. Rather, greater risk of salmonellosis was realized from lightly contaminated chickens when they were temperature-abused, undercooked, and consumed by someone from the high risk population.*

INTRODUCTION

Risk assessment of microbial hazards in food involves four components: hazard identification, exposure assessment (i.e., dose consumed), dose-response assessment (i.e., infectious dose), and risk characterization (i.e., probability of infection) (Rose *et al.* 1995). Epidemiological studies indicate that *Salmonella spp.* are a primary microbial hazard associated with poultry products (Bryan and Doyle 1995). The risk or probability of acquiring salmonellosis from consumption of poultry products depends on the *Salmonella* load of the poultry product at consumption, the amount of poultry product consumed, and the infectious dose of *Salmonella*. In turn, the infectious dose of *Salmonella* is a function of the virulence of the *Salmonella* strain, the composition of the food, and the physiological state of the consumer.

With the advent of computer software programs, such as @Risk™, that perform simulations of models created in common spreadsheet programs, such as Excel™, it is now possible to create computer models that predict the risk of salmonellosis from poultry products produced by specified farm-to-table scenarios (Whiting and Buchanan 1997). The present paper describes and demonstrates a simulation model that assesses the risk of acquiring salmonellosis from consumption of chicken. The model simulates the distribution, preparation, and consumption of 1,000 chickens and was designed to determine the relationship between the level of *Salmonella* contamination of chickens leaving the processing plant and the risk of salmonellosis for consumers who ate the chickens.

APPROACH

Model Design

Figure 1 shows the layout of the risk assessment model. The model was constructed in an Excel™ spreadsheet and was simulated using @Risk™ (Palisade Corp., Newfield, NY). The model consisted of nine nodes. The first three nodes in the model were a series of pathogen events that modeled the change in *Salmonella* load of the chickens as they moved from the processing plant exit to consumption. Node four modeled direct consumption of *Salmonella* from cooked chicken, node five modeled indirect consumption of *Salmonella* from handling the raw chicken, node six calculated the total dose of *Salmonella* consumed, node seven modeled the infectious dose of consumers in the normal population, node eight modeled the infectious dose of consumers in the high risk population, and node nine calculated the probability of salmonellosis for each consumption event.

The variability of *Salmonella* load among chickens in the flock and the variability of chicken consumption and infectious dose among consumers were modeled using a combination of probability distributions. A Discrete distribution was used to model the incidence of these nodes, whereas a Pert distribution was used to model the extent of these nodes. A Pert distribution is a continuous distribution that is defined by three values: minimum, most likely, and maximum. The shape of the Pert distribution can vary from normal to log normal depending on the values used to define it.

	Extent				
Node	Incidence	Minimum	Most Likely	Maximum	Output
Raw Chicken	20%	0 log	1.0 log	3.0 log	7
Temperature Abuse	20%	0.1 log	0.5 log	3.0 log	335
Cooking	20%	-2.0 log	-1.5 log	-1 log	0
Consumption, Direct	100%	15%	25%	50%	0
Consumption, Indirect	25%	1%	2%	5%	8.7
Dose Consumed					8.7
Infectious Dose, Normal	80%	500	750	1000	
Infectious Dose, High Risk	20%	50	200	350	142
Probability of Salmonellosis					6.2%

FIG. 1. SIMULATION MODEL FOR ASSESSING THE PROBABILITY OF ACQUIRING SALMONELLOSIS FROM CONSUMPTION OF CHICKEN
Output results are for iteration 844 and are expressed as *Salmonella*/bird.

During simulation of the current model (Fig. 1), @Risk randomly sampled the Pert distribution for each node as a function of their incidence and used the random numbers selected to calculate the outputs of the model. The model was simulated once using Latin hypercube sampling and 1,000 iterations. The following outputs were calculated by the model: (1) the *Salmonella* load of raw chicken at the processing plant exit; (2) the *Salmonella* load of raw chicken after temperature abuse during distribution and meal preparation; (3) the *Salmonella* load of cooked chicken; (4) the dose of *Salmonella* consumed directly from cooked chicken; (5) the dose of *Salmonella* consumed indirectly from handling of raw chickens; (6) the total dose of *Salmonella* consumed; (7) the infectious dose of *Salmonella*; and (8) the probability of acquiring salmonellosis from consumption of chicken. The results of iteration 844 from the simulation are shown in Fig. 1 as an example of the output generated by the model.

RESULTS AND DISCUSSION

Salmonella Load of Raw Chicken at the Processing Plant Exit

The model (Fig. 1) was defined such that 20% or 200 of the 1,000 chickens simulated were contaminated with *Salmonella* at the plant exit. The extent of contamination of the 200 *Salmonella*-positive chickens was modeled by a Pert distribution defined by a minimum value of 0 log or 1 *Salmonella*, a most likely value of 1 log or 10 *Salmonella*, and a maximum value of 3 log or 1,000 *Salmonella*. During simulation of the model, @Risk randomly sampled the Pert distribution to determine the level of contamination of each of the 200 *Salmonella*-positive chickens. The level of contamination ranged from 1 to 953 *Salmonella* per bird (Fig. 2) which is in agreement with published data (Surkiewicz *et al.* 1969).

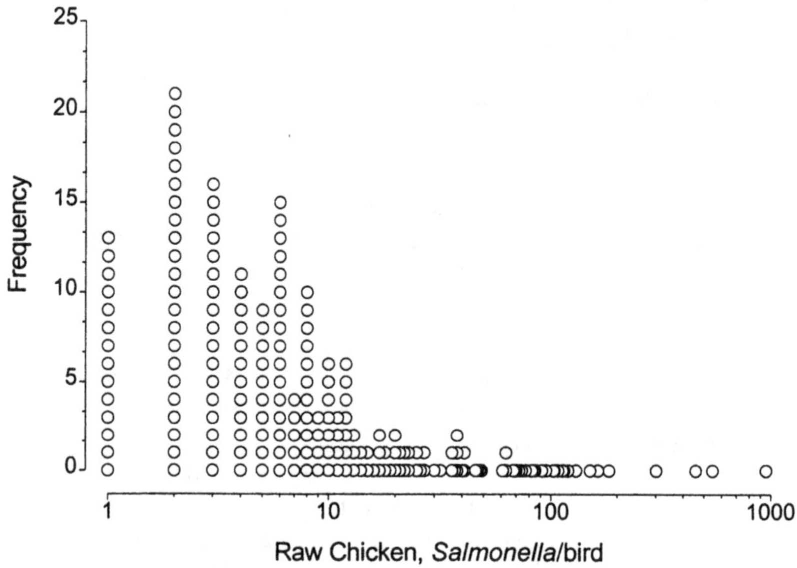

FIG. 2. FREQUENCY DISTRIBUTION OF THE *SALMONELLA* LOAD OF 200 *SALMONELLA*-POSITIVE CHICKENS AS THEY LEFT THE PROCESSING PLANT

Salmonella Load of Raw Chicken after Temperature Abuse

The second node in the model (Fig. 1) simulated temperature abuse that resulted in growth of *Salmonella* on the chickens during distribution and meal preparation. Similar to contamination of the raw chickens, temperature abuse was modeled by considering its incidence and extent. Although a consumer survey by Worsfold and Griffith (1997) indicated that 45% of consumers temperature abuse their food during transport, the incidence of temperature abuse during distribution and meal preparation was set at 20% in the current model and the variation of the extent of *Salmonella* growth on the chickens during temperature abuse was defined by a Pert distribution with a minimum value of a 0.1 log cycle increase, a most likely value of a 0.5-log cycle increase, and a maximum value of a 3.0 log cycle increase. Results of the simulation indicated that of the 200 *Salmonella*-positive chickens at the plant exit only 33 underwent temperature abuse (i.e., those circular symbols in Fig. 3 above the circular symbols that form a straight line) during distribution and meal preparation. The level of contamination of the 200 *Salmonella*-positive chickens after temperature abuse ranged from 1 to 11,814 *Salmonella* per bird (Fig. 3).

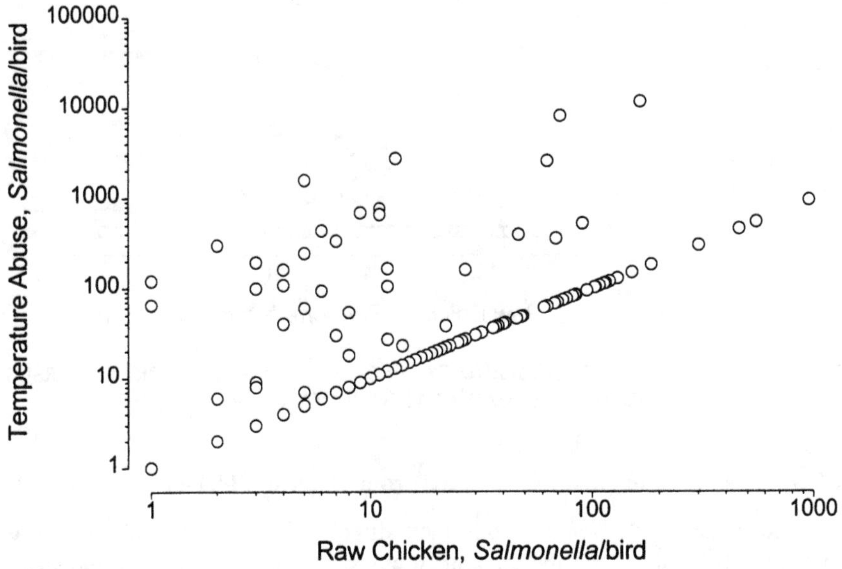

FIG. 3. SCATTER PLOT OF THE *SALMONELLA* LOAD OF RAW CHICKENS AFTER TEMPERATURE ABUSE DURING DISTRIBUTION AND MEAL PREPARATION VERSUS THEIR *SALMONELLA* LOAD AT THE PROCESSING PLANT EXIT

Salmonella Load of Cooked Chicken

The third node in the model (Fig. 1) simulated the impact of cooking on the number of *Salmonella* consumed. Results of a survey by Worsfold and Griffith (1997) indicated that 15% of consumers undercook their food. In the current model, cooking was defined such that 20% of the chickens were undercooked resulting in 1 to 10% survival of the contaminating *Salmonella*. It was assumed that the other 80% of the chickens were properly cooked resulting in no survival of *Salmonella*. Results of the simulation indicated that of the 200 chickens contaminated with *Salmonella* at the plant exit only nine were undercooked resulting in survival of between 1 and 445 *Salmonella* per bird (Fig. 4).

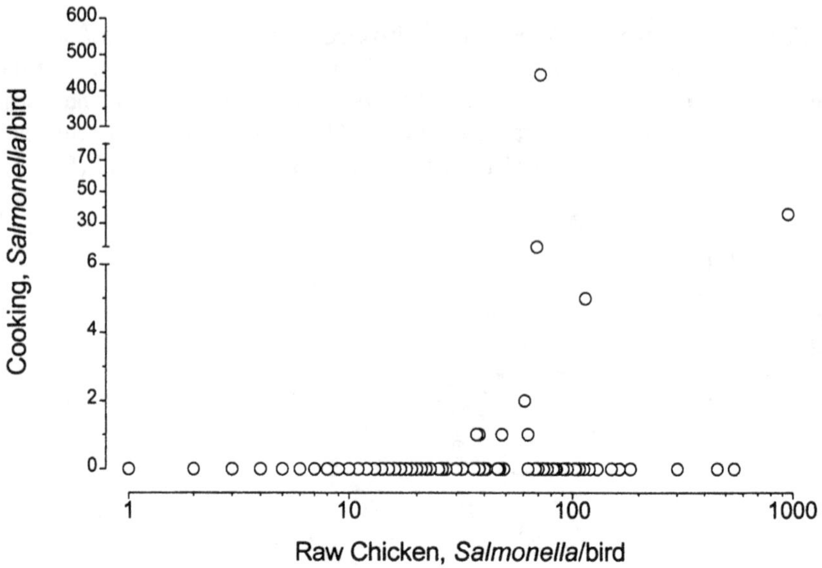

FIG. 4. SCATTER PLOT OF THE *SALMONELLA* LOAD OF COOKED CHICKENS VERSUS THEIR *SALMONELLA* LOAD AT THE PROCESSING PLANT EXIT

Direct Dose of *Salmonella* Consumed from Cooked Chicken

The dose of *Salmonella* consumed directly from cooked chicken was calculated by multiplying the amount of chicken consumed by the *Salmonella* load of the chicken after cooking. The variation in the amount of a chicken consumed was modeled by a Pert distribution with a minimum value of 15%, a most likely value of 25%, and a maximum value of 50%. Of the 200 *Salmonella*-positive chickens at the plant exit only nine were still contaminated after cooking and thus, resulted in direct consumption of *Salmonella* by consumers. The direct dose of *Salmonella* consumed from these nine chickens ranged from 0.3 to 102.7 *Salmonella*/bird (Fig. 5). The direct dose of *Salmonella* consumed was expressed as a fraction because it was a probability that was calculated by assuming that the contaminating *Salmonella* were uniformly distributed on the chicken.

Indirect Dose of *Salmonella* Consumed from Handling of Raw Chicken

The average amount of chicken consumed by consumers was 25%. Thus, each chicken was consumed on average by four consumers. It was assumed that one of these four consumers was the food handler who prepared the chicken for consumption. Thus, the incidence of indirect consumption of *Salmonella* by consumers was 25% (Fig. 1). The extent of indirect consumption of *Salmonella* by food handlers was defined by a Pert distribution with a minimum value of 1%, a most likely value of 2%, and a maximum value of 5%. Results of the simulation indicated that of the 200 *Salmonella*-positive chickens at the plant exit, 61 resulted in ingestion of *Salmonella* by food handlers. The dose of *Salmonella* ingested by food handlers ranged from 0.015 to 310 *Salmonella* (Fig. 6) and was calculated by multiplying the *Salmonella* load after temperature abuse by the percentage of *Salmonella* ingested by food handlers.

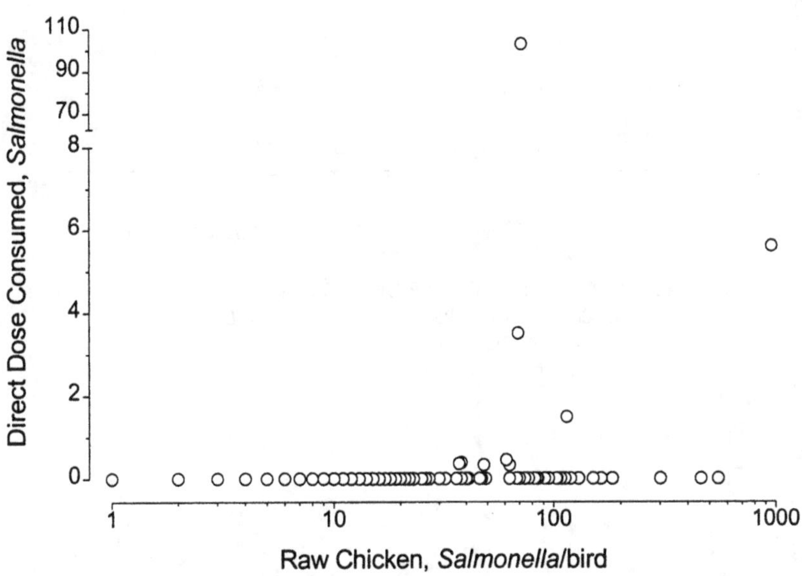

FIG. 5. SCATTER PLOT OF THE DOSE OF *SALMONELLA* CONSUMED FROM COOKED CHICKENS VERSUS THEIR *SALMONELLA* LOAD AT THE PROCESSING PLANT EXIT

Total Dose of *Salmonella* Consumed

The total dose of *Salmonella* consumed was obtained by adding the dose of *Salmonella* consumed directly from the cooked chicken to the dose of *Salmonella* consumed from handling the raw chicken. Of the 200 *Salmonella*-positive chickens at the plant exit, none of the nine chickens still contaminated after cooking were consumed by food handlers. Thus, the total number of chickens that resulted in a dose of *Salmonella* consumed was 70. The total dose consumed from these 70 chickens ranged from 0.015 to 310 *Salmonella* (Fig. 7).

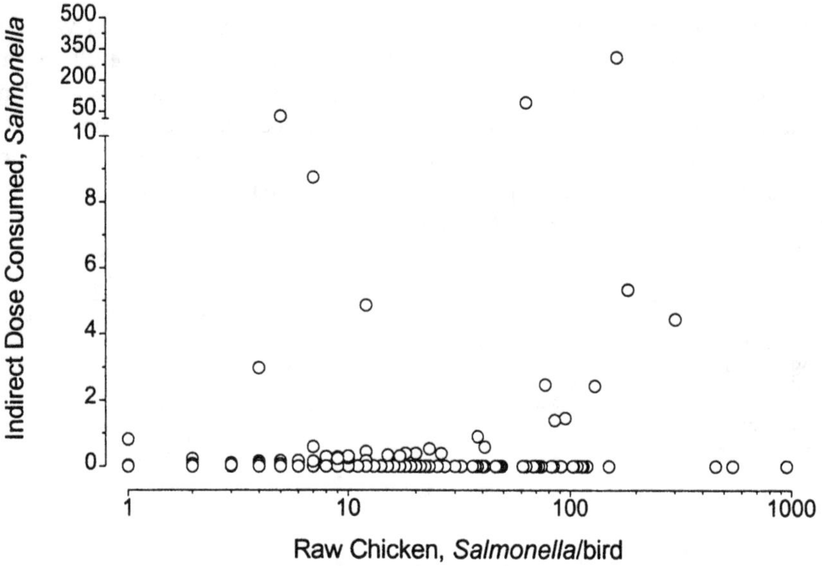

FIG. 6. SCATTER PLOT OF THE DOSE OF *SALMONELLA* CONSUMED FROM HANDLING RAW CHICKENS VERSUS THEIR *SALMONELLA* LOAD AT THE PROCESSING PLANT EXIT

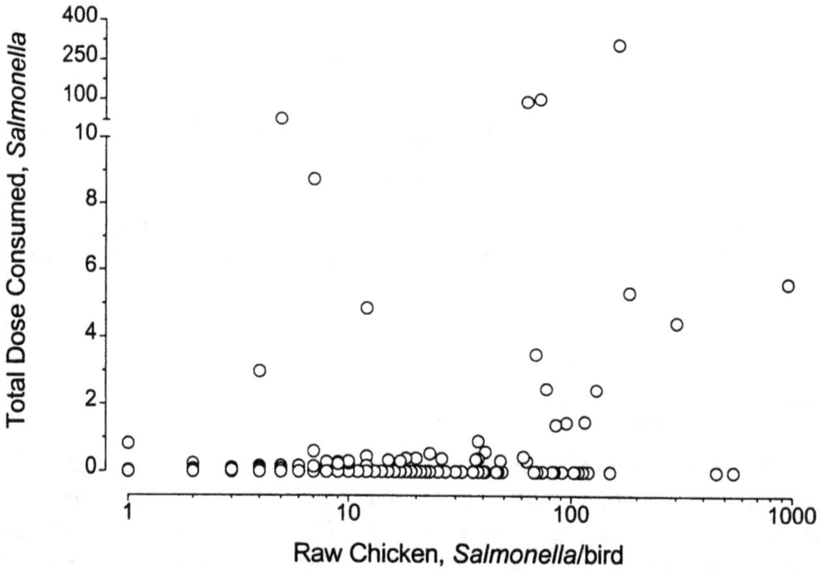

FIG. 7. SCATTER PLOT OF THE TOTAL DOSE OF *SALMONELLA* CONSUMED FROM CONSUMPTION AND HANDLING OF CHICKENS VERSUS THEIR *SALMONELLA* LOAD AT THE PROCESSING PLANT EXIT

Infectious Dose

Infectious dose was defined such that 80% of consumers were from the normal population and 20% were from the high risk (i.e., immunocompromised) population. The Pert distribution for infectious dose of individuals in the normal population was defined by a minimum value of 500 *Salmonella*, a most likely value of 750 *Salmonella*, and a maximum value of 1,000 *Salmonella* (Fig. 1). The Pert distribution for infectious dose of individuals in the high risk population was defined by a minimum value of 50 *Salmonella*, a most likely value of 200 *Salmonella*, and a maximum value of 350 *Salmonella* (Fig. 1). The values used to define infectious dose in the model are consistent with those reported for *Salmonella* which range from 10^1 to 10^9 depending on the strain of *Salmonella* and food vehicle (Blaser and Newman 1982). For the 200 *Salmonella*-positive chickens at the plant exit, Fig. 8 shows the random selection of infectious dose for each of the consumers who ate those chickens.

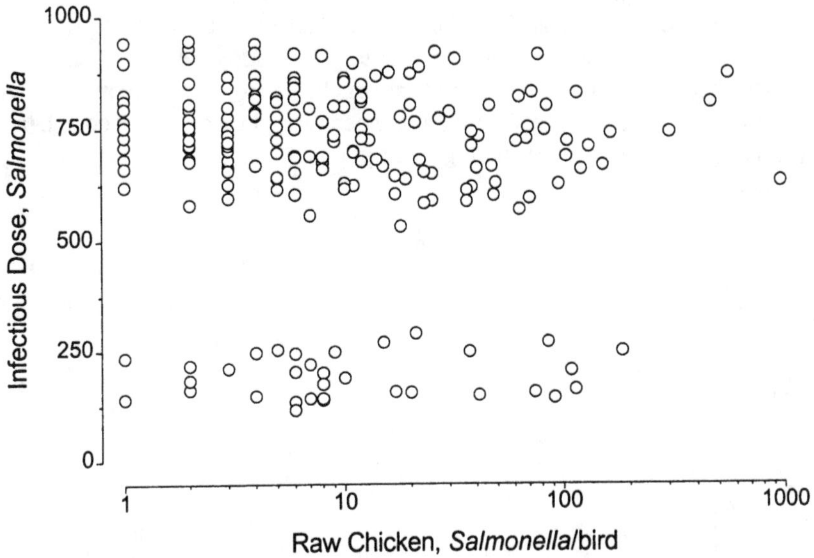

FIG. 8. SCATTER PLOT OF THE INFECTIOUS DOSE OF *SALMONELLA* FOR CONSUMERS IN THE NORMAL (UPPER CLUSTER) AND HIGH RISK (LOWER CLUSTER) POPULATIONS VERSUS THE *SALMONELLA* LOAD OF THE CHICKENS AT THE PROCESSING PLANT EXIT

Probability of Acquiring Salmonellosis from Consumption of Chicken

Finally, the model calculated the probability of acquiring salmonellosis for each of the 1,000 chickens simulated using the following equation:

$$P = \text{IF (D/I} > 1, 1, \text{D/I)} * 100$$

where *P* was the probability of acquiring salmonellosis in %, *D* was the total dose of *Salmonella* consumed, *I* was the infectious dose of *Salmonella*, and the statement read that IF the ratio of *D* to *I* was greater than one then *P* was one otherwise *P* was the ratio of *D* to *I*. This calculation assumed that one *Salmonella* was capable of causing an infection and that infectious dose was the dose of *Salmonella* consumed that resulted in a 100% probability of salmonellosis. This calculation of the probability of salmonellosis for each consumption event was very similar to the exponential dose-response model used by others (Haas 1983; Rose *et al.* 1995) except that it was assumed that the probability of salmonellosis increased linearly rather than exponentially as a function of dose consumed and infectious dose.

Of the 1,000 chickens simulated only 70 or 7% posed a risk of salmonellosis. The probability of salmonellosis from these 70 chickens ranged from 0.0018 to 42.1% (Fig. 9). In addition, results in Fig. 9 showed that highly (i.e., > 100 *Salmonella*/bird) contaminated chickens at the plant exit did not necessarily pose greater risk of salmonellosis than lightly (i.e., < 10 *Salmonella*/bird) contaminated chickens. Rather, greater risk of salmonellosis from lightly contaminated chickens was realized when they were temperature abused, undercooked, and consumed by someone from the high risk population.

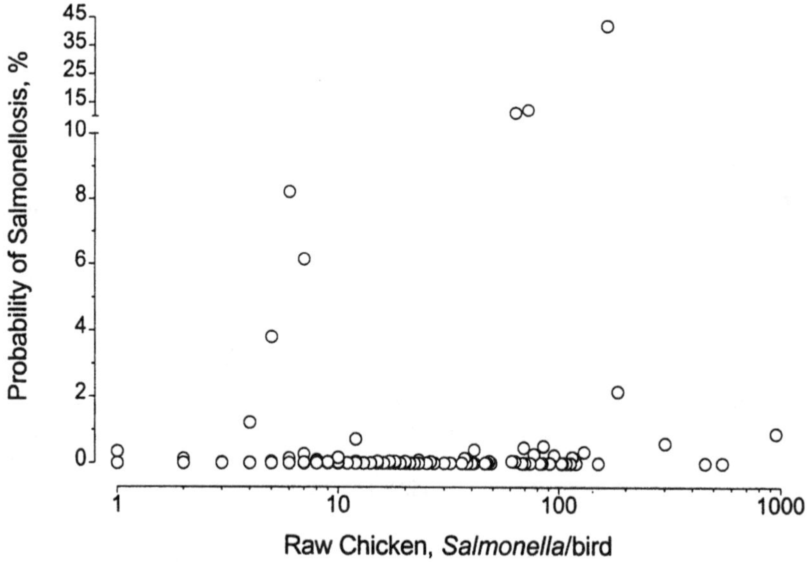

FIG. 9. SCATTER PLOT OF THE PROBABILITY OF ACQUIRING SALMONELLOSIS VERSUS THE *SALMONELLA* LOAD OF THE CHICKENS AS THEY LEFT THE PROCESSING PLANT

CONCLUSION

A simulation model was designed to determine the relationship between the level of *Salmonella* contamination of chickens at the processing plant exit and the risk of salmonellosis in consumers. Results of the model simulation indicated that greater risk of salmonellosis can be realized from lightly (i.e., < 10 *Salmonella*/bird) than heavily (i.e., > 100 *Salmonella*/bird) contaminated chickens. Thus, current attempts by the poultry industry to lower the incidence of *Salmonella* contamination of raw poultry are justified.

REFERENCES

BLASER, M.J. and NEWMAN, L.S. 1982. A review of human salmonellosis: I. Infective dose. Rev. Infect. Dis. *4*, 1096–1106.

BRYAN, F.L. and DOYLE, M.P. 1995. Health risks and consequences of *Salmonella* and *Campylobacter jejuni* in raw poultry. J. Food Prot. *58*, 326-344.

HAAS, C.N. 1983. Estimation of risk due to low doses of microorganisms: a comparison of alternative methodologies. Am. J. Epidemiol. *118*, 573–582.

ROSE, J.B., HAAS, C.N. and GERBA, C.P. 1995. Linking microbiological criteria for foods with quantitative risk assessment. J. Food Safety *15*, 121–132.

SURKIEWICZ, B.F., JOHNSTON, R.W., MORAN, A.B. and KRUMM, G. W. 1969. A bacteriological survey of chicken eviscerating plants. Food Technol. *23*, 80–85.

WHITING, R.C. and BUCHANAN, R.L. 1997. Development of a quantitative risk assessment model for Salmonella enteritidis in pasteurized liquid eggs. Int. J. Food Microbiol. *36*, 111–125.

WORSFOLD, D. and GRIFFITH, C.J. 1997. Assessment of the standard of consumer food safety behavior. J. Food Prot. *60*, 399–406.

CHAPTER 10

FACTORS INVOLVED IN RECENT OUTBREAKS OF *ESCHERICHIA COLI* O157:H7 IN SCOTLAND AND RECOMMENDATIONS FOR ITS CONTROL

HUGH PENNINGTON

Aberdeen Royal Hospital
NHS Trust
Aberdeen, Scotland

ABSTRACT

This paper describes an outbreak of E. coli *O157:H7 that occurred in central Scotland. Edipemiological and microbiological evidence has indicated that the outbreak was comprised of several separate but related incidents, relating to the lunch (attended by around 100 people) held in Wishaw Parish Church Hall, a birthday party held in a public house on November 23, 1996 and retail sales in Lanarkshire and Forth Valley. All isolates of* E. coli *O157:H7 from individuals in the outbreak belonged to phage type 2 and possessed the verocytotoxin gene VT2. Two hundred sixty-two of these isolates have been subjected to pulsed-field gel electrophoresis (PFGE): all had indistinguishable profiles. There were 496 cases in total. There have been 20 deaths (all adults) associated with the outbreak, the highest number of deaths associated with an outbreak of* E. coli *O157:H7 infection in the world. Of these, 8 people had attended the luncheon served at Wishaw Old Parish Church on November 27, 1996. The age range of those who died was 69 to 93 years. The outbreak was investigated by the Pennington Group who concluded that the circumstances of the central Scotland outbreak, and the inevitable uncertainties that may surround outbreaks generally, provide strong justification for the precautionary, preventative measures proposed and the recommendations made.*

INTRODUCTION

At this time legal constraints prevent a description or debate in any detail of the full circumstances of the central Scotland outbreak or the individual roles and actions of those involved in it. What can be discussed briefly is the course and scale of the outbreak and some of the key facts, statistics and issues associated with it in order to help set the context for the recommendations of the Pennington Expert Group. This account is based on the final report, published in April 1998.

Background

The start of a food poisoning outbreak caused by *E. coli* O157:H7 was signalled on the afternoon of Friday, November 22, 1996 when the Public Health Department of Lanarkshire Health Board was informed of several cases of infection (some of which had been confirmed by microbiological testing) in residents of Wishaw in central Scotland.

By the evening of November 22, 1996, histories had been obtained from 9 confirmed or suspected cases. Indications were that 8 of these 9 had consumed food obtained, either directly or at a church lunch, from J. Barr and Son, Butchers, of Wishaw. The possibility of other common exposures could not at this stage be excluded, as a significant proportion of the population of Wishaw probably patronised J. Barr and Son in any one week. Although outwardly a small, local butcher with adjacent bakery shop, the business was involved at the time of the outbreak in a substantial wholesale and retail trade involving the production and distribution of raw and cooked meats and bakery products from the Wishaw premises. It employed about 40 people, many on a part-time basis.

The distribution chain of meat and meat products from J. Barr and Son was complex and it took some time for the details to be unravelled by a painstaking investigation of the company's records. That caused delays in relation to the public identification of some of the outlets involved or potentially involved in the outbreak. Some 85 outlets throughout central Scotland were eventually identified as being supplied by the company.

As indicated by the epidemic curve for the outbreak, the number of cases of suspected or confirmed infection increased dramatically (Fig. 1). Epidemiological and microbiological evidence has indicated that the outbreak comprised of several separate but related incidents relating to a lunch (attended by around 100 people) held in Wishaw Parish Church Hall, a birthday party held in a public house on November 23, 1996, and retail sales in Lanarkshire and Forth Valley. All isolates of *E. coli* O157:H7 from individuals in the outbreak belonged to phage type 2 and possessed the verocytotoxin gene VT2. Two hundred and sixty-two of these isolates have been subjected to pulsed-field gel electrophoresis (PFGE): all had indistinguishable profiles. The final number of cases is shown in Table 1.

The outbreak put great pressures on local health resources. Thus a clinic in Wishaw carried out batches of tests on some 969 people with diarrhoea, and 127 people were hospitalized, 13 requiring dialysis. Twenty-seven people were diagnosed as having either the haemolytic uraemic syndrome or thrombotic

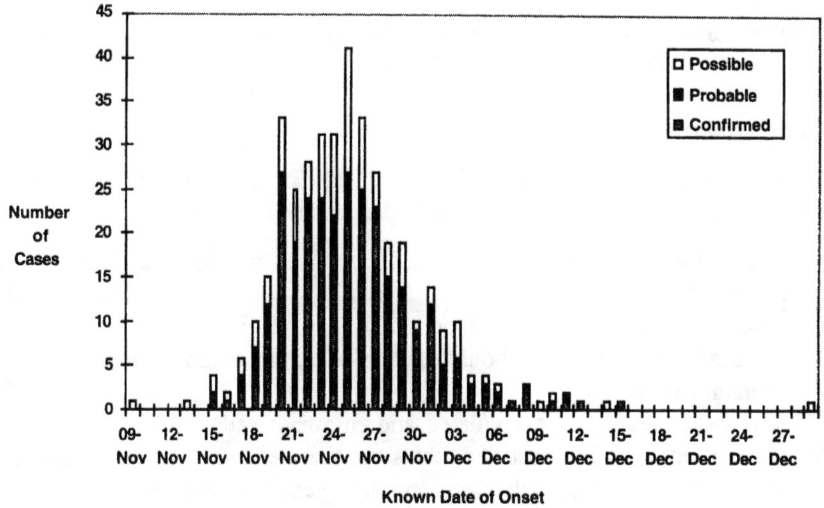

FIG. 1. EPIDEMIC CURVE FOR *E. COLI* O157:H7 OUTBREAK IN CENTRAL SCOTLAND SHOWING THE DATE OF THE ONSET OF DIARRHOEA

TABLE 1.
NUMBERS OF CONFIRMED, PROBABLE OR POSSIBLE CASES FROM AN OUTBREAK OF *E.COLI* O157:H7 IN SCOTLAND

	All Scotland	Lanarkshire	Forth Valley	Greater Lothian	Glasgow
Confirmed[1]	272	195	73	4	0
Probable[2]	60	50	10	0	0
Probable[3]	164	128	35	0	1
Total	496	373	118	4	1

Note: Patient with *E. coli* O157 identified in their stool, irrespective of clinical history.

[1]Confirmed case:

[2]Probable case: Patient with bloody diarrhoea and positive serology.

[3]Possible case: Patient who has non-bloody diarrhoea with positive serology *or* someone who has no symptoms with positive serology *or* patient who has bloody diarrhoea without positive serology.

thrombocytopaenia purpura. There have been 20 deaths (all adults) associated with the outbreak, the highest number of deaths associated with an outbreak of *E. coli* O157:H7 infection in the world. Of these, 8 people had attended the luncheon served at Wishaw Old Parish Church on November 17, 1996. The age range of those who died was 69 to 93 years.

Issues Arising

The central Scotland outbreak caused the Expert Group to examine a number of general issues and questions, particularly:

(1) how and why fresh meat becomes contaminated with *E. coli* O157:H7 in the first place;
(2) the likely distribution in the food chain;
(3) the measures that can and should be taken to minimise contamination/cross-contamination;
(4) how these measures are regulated and enforced; and
(5) once an outbreak has occurred, the steps that need to be taken to manage and control it, and the adequacy and arrangements necessary.

The potential for contamination/cross-contamination with the organism, its virulence and the very severe effects it can have on particularly vulnerable groups of the community were tragically underlined by the outbreak. Of particular significance is the issue of asymptomatic excretion of the organism, which may have very substantial implications in terms of the potential for the spread of infection and outbreak management and control. The Pennington Group concluded that the circumstances of the central Scotland outbreak, and the inevitable uncertainties that may surround outbreaks generally, provide strong justification for the precautionary, preventative measures proposed and the recommendations made.

E. coli O157:H7

E. coli O157:H7 was first identified as a cause of human illness in 1982 in patients affected in 2 outbreaks of bloody diarrhoea in the USA, both associated with eating undercooked hamburgers. There have since been numerous and increasing reports world-wide of infection with the organism (Armstrong *et al.* 1996). This may be due in part to improved surveillance and methods of detection, but it is generally accepted that increases in the rate of infection with the organism are real rather than due simply to improved ascertainment.

Outbreaks in the UK/Scotland

Most outbreaks in the UK have affected fewer than 10 people and have been associated with the consumption of a variety of foods including minced beef (including hamburgers), milk, yoghurt, cheese and water. Prior to the central Scotland outbreak, the largest recorded outbreak was in West Lothian in

1994 associated with the consumption of contaminated pasteurised milk, when more than 100 people were affected and a child died.

The number of laboratory-confirmed cases of human infection with *E. coli* O157:H7 in Scotland were reported to the Scottish Centre for Infection and Environmental Health in Glasgow, and in England and Wales to the Public Health Laboratory Service's Communicable Disease Surveillance Centre, London. The respective rates of infection per 100,000 population, since 1990 are shown in Table 2. The 1994 and 1996 figures for Scotland are, obviously, heavily influenced by the effects of the West Lothian and central Scotland outbreaks.

TABLE 2.
NUMBERS OF LABORATORY CONFIRMED CASES OF *E. COLI* O157:H7 IN SCOTLAND AND ENGLAND AND WALES AND THE RATES OF INFECTION FROM 1990 TO 1996

	Scotland		England & Wales	
	No. of Cases	Rate	No. of Cases	Rate
1990	173	3.39	250	0.49
1991	202	3.96	361	0.71
1992	115	2.25	470	0.92
1993	119	2.32	385	0.75
1994	242	4.71	411	0.80
1995	247	4.8	792	1.52
1996	488*	9.5**	660*	1.26**

*Provisional
**Projected rates based on 1995 mid-year population estimates

Because of the general difficulties in identification of the organism, recent improvements in detection methods and differences in, for example, surveillance practices, it is difficult to make definitive, detailed comparisons annually or among different parts of the UK; However the underlying rate of infection in Scotland, per 100,000 of population, is substantially higher than for England and Wales (around 4 times). The reasons for this are unclear.

How Infection Occurs

E. coli O157:H7 exists in a wide range of animals, both wild and domestic. It is generally accepted that its main animal reservoir is the rumens and intestines of cattle and sheep (Anon 1997a).

The organism is excreted and can exist in animal manure or slurry, which could be a source of environmental or water contamination or direct contamination of food such as vegetables; however, most of the evidence for this is circumstantial. It seems likely that there can be animal-to-animal infection/reinfection. There is good evidence that it is transferred to animal carcasses through contamination from faecal matter during the slaughter process. Many early outbreaks were associated with the consumption of undercooked hamburgers. There have also been documented cases attributed to other foods such as milk, cheese and apple juice. In a recent large Japanese outbreak, radishes were identified as a possible source of the infection (Anon. 1995).

The organism survives well in frozen storage so freezing cannot be relied upon to kill it. It is killed by heating, but can survive if food is not properly cooked (as in the case of hamburgers mentioned above). If appropriate hygiene measures are not taken, there can also be cross-contamination between raw meat carrying the organism and cooked or ready-to-eat foods. It is relatively tolerant to acidic conditions (compared, for example, to *Salmonella*).

Human infection may occur as a result of direct contact with animals, from contamination with their faeces, or through consumption of contaminated food or water. It may also spread directly from person-to-person by faecal-oral transmission. The latter is, obviously, a particular potential problem in institutions such as nursing homes, day-care centres, hospitals, and in places where pre-school children meet which underlines the need for good personal hygiene and meticulous attention to procedures designed to prevent cross-infection. Cases may be related to outbreaks or may be sporadic, i.e., isolated and apparently unrelated to other cases). The role of asymptomatic food handlers in outbreaks is unclear but may be important in light of the low infectious dose (Armstrong *et al.* 1997).

Detection and Identification

Despite improvements in surveillance and testing techniques, the organism remains more difficult to detect and identify accurately than other important foodborne bacterial pathogens. *E. coli* O157:H7 does not generally cause illness in animals and there is no reason for farmers to seek to identify the presence of the organism in their animals. In any event it appears to be excreted only intermittently. It has been difficult to identify in foods and although techniques have improved over the years, rates of detection are still unsatisfactory. This is due in part to the low levels of the organism which occur in food. The most sensitive techniques for identifying the organism in food are complex and sophisticated, requiring special equipment and expertise that is not generally available (Anon. 1995).

SUMMARY OF RECOMMENDATIONS OF THE PENNINGTON GROUP

Early in the outbreak, on the 28th of November, 1996, the Secretary of State for Scotland asked that an expert group be convened "to examine the circumstances which led to the outbreak in the central belt of Scotland and to advise him on the implications for food safety and the general lessons to be learned". The recommendations in the final report, which have been accepted by the Government are summarized below (Anon. 1997b).

Farms and Livestock

There should be an education/awareness programme for farm workers, repeated and updated periodically as appropriate, to ensure they are aware:

(1) of the existence, potential prevalence and nature of *E. coli* O157:H7;
(2) of the potential for the spread of infection on farms, notably from faecal material, and of the consequent need for scrupulous personal hygiene;
(3) of the need for care in the use of untreated slurry or manure; and
(4) of the absolute requirement for the presentation of animals in an appropriate, clean condition for slaughter.

All of this must be backed up by rigorous enforcement.

Slaughterhouses

(1) Good practice in slaughterhouses must be identified and promoted by Industry with the help and support of government departments, particularly in the areas the presentation of clean cattle and of hide and intestine removal.
(2) Abattoir workers should be trained in good hygiene practice during slaughter and enforcement should concentrate on slaughter and subsequent handling of carcasses.
(3) The Hazard Analysis and Critical Control Point system should be enshrined in the legislation governing slaughterhouses and the transportation of carcasses and meat. Meanwhile, enforcers and the trade should ensure that HACCP principles are observed.
(4) Further consideration should be given, involving the industry and consumer interests, to the potential use and benefits of end-process treatments such as steam pasteurisation.

Meat Production Premises and Butcher's Shops

(1) HACCP (i.e. the approach and all 7 principles) should be adopted by all food businesses to ensure food safety. While this is being negotiated into European Union and domestic legislation, implementation and enforcement of the HACCP principles contained in existing legislation should be accelerated.
(2) Pending HACCP implementation, selective licensing arrangements for premises not covered by the Meat Products (Hygiene) Regulations 1994 should be introduced by new regulations.
(3) The licensing arrangements should include appropriate requirements for the documentation of hazard analysis, labelling and record-keeping to facilitate product recall, and temperature control and monitoring. In relation to training, there should be a requirement for all food handlers to have undertaken at least a basic food training course and for all supervisory staff (and those who run small, one-person operations) to be trained to at least intermediate level. In addition the licence should cover matters relating to the suitability of premises, equipment and hygiene practices to a level equivalent to that required by the 1994 Regulations.

In Relation to the Physical Separation Requirements of Licensing

(1) There should be separation, in storage, production, sale and display, between raw meat and unwrapped cooked meat/meat products and other ready-to-eat foods. This should include the use of separate refrigerators and production equipment, utensils and wherever possible, staff.
(2) Where the use of separate staff cannot be achieved, alternative standards (such as the completion and implementation by the operator of a HACCP program or the provision and use of additional facilities, e.g., for hand washing in the serving area might be regarded as sufficient to permit the award of a licence).
(3) Where neither can be achieved, the premises concerned should not be permitted to sell both raw and unwrapped cooked meat/cooked meat products, although they may be permitted to sell pre-wrapped cooked/ready-to-eat meat products prepared elsewhere and brought in for that purpose.

Point of Consumption

(1) Food hygiene training should be provided wherever possible within the primary and secondary school curriculum.
(2) Guidance and education about food handling and hygiene should be included in all food and catering education and training courses and should be reinforced through periodic advertising and awareness initiatives.

(3) Steps should be taken by local authorities to encourage the adoption of HACCP principles in nonregistered premises where there is catering for functions for groups of people involving the serving of more than just tea, coffee and confectionery goods.

(4) Employers should ensure that the food handlers, in particular those working with vulnerable groups and/or in sensitive areas such as nursing homes and day-care centres, are aware of and implement good hygiene practice. They should be trained in food hygiene at least to the basic and preferably intermediate level.

Enforcement

(1) The Government should give a clear policy lead on the need for the enforcement of food safety measures and the accelerated implementation of HACCP.

(2) The government and local authority should ensure that there are available suitable and adequate Environmental Health Officer skills and resources to address enforcement and education/awareness issues.

(3) The Government should consider earmarking local authority funds for these purposes.

(4) Local authorities should designate an environmental health officer, with appropriate training, experience and expertise, to head food safety within the authority.

Recommendation on surveillance, research and outbreak control were also made.

REFERENCES

ANON. 1997a. Prevention and Control of Enterohaemorrhagic *Escherichia coli* (EHEC) Infections. Report of a WHO Consultation, Geneva, Switzerland, 28 April - 1 May 1997. WHO, 1997.

ANON. 1997b. The Pennington Group: Report on the Circumstances Leading to the 1996 Outbreak of Infection with *E. coli* O157 in Central Scotland, the Implications for Food Safety and the Lessons to be Learned. 1997. Edinburgh: The Stationery Office.

ANON. 1995. Advisory Committee on the Microbial Safety of Food. Report on Verocytotoxin-Producing Escherichia coli. 1995. HMSO, London.

ARMSTRONG, G.L., HOLLINGSWORGH, J. and MORRIS, J.G. 1996. Emerging foodborne pathogens: *Escherichia coli* O157:H7 as a model of entry of a new pathogen in the food supply of the developed world. Epidemiologic Rev. *18*, 29–51.

CHAPTER 11

SOURCES OF CONTAMINATION DURING SLAUGHTER AND MEASURES FOR CONTROL

J. J. SHERIDAN

Teagasc, The National Food Centre
Dunsinea, Castleknock, Dublin 15, Ireland

ABSTRACT

This paper is concerned with processes and procedures involved in the contamination of beef, lamb and pork carcasses during slaughter. The hides of beef and the fleece of sheep are major sources of carcass contamination. The spread of pathogens from beef hides to the carcass, operatives and surfaces in the abattoir is demonstrated. Efforts to clean the hide of cattle and the fleece of sheep are outlined, with reference to the success of these treatments in reducing carcass contamination. The effect of bringing very dirty or dungy animals to slaughter is considered in terms of the effect on carcass contamination after slaughter. The influence of tying the bung (or rectum) in reducing carcass contamination is discussed, as is the use of plastic bags as an additional control in preventing pathogen spread on pig carcasses. The relationship of this revised procedure in reducing the occurrence of yersiniosis in Norway is shown. The use of a commercially automated system to tie beef bungs is discussed in relation to reducing carcass contamination. A comparison between the removal of faecal contamination on carcasses by trimming or using a new steam-vacuumized system is presented. The effect of preevisceration washing of beef carcasses is described and the rationale relating to bacterial removal using this treatment is discussed. The influence of evisceration as a source of carcass contamination is demonstrated in relation to sheep slaughter. The processes of carcass decontamination using washing with water at different temperatures, steam pasteurization and hot lactic acid are compared in relation to their ability to remove bacteria from beef carcass surfaces. Finally, the effect of line speed and the impact of technology advances on beef and sheep carcass contamination is reviewed.

INTRODUCTION

Most sectors of the food industry face a major and continuing challenge in trying to limit the extent to which food products become contaminated with pathogenic bacteria during primary processing. Nowhere is this more apparent than in meat processing, where the production of meat from live animals presents many opportunities for contamination with a range of pathogens. In recent years the meat industry and regulatory authorities have attempted to limit the presence of pathogens on carcasses by the application of Hazard Analysis and Critical Control Points (HACCP) systems within meat plants. These are designed to assist in the management and control of the slaughter process by identifying the critical control points where contamination can occur and specifying actions that can be taken to improve the hygienic status of the carcass.

This paper considers the different points on the line where intervention can affect carcass hygiene and examines the impact of new process efficiency or safety technologies on carcass hygiene. While carcass decontamination is important in this context and is considered here, it is not considered in a comprehensive way. It also assesses the long-term effects of the gradual introduction of new technology and considers the impact of other process variables, such as line speed, on carcass hygiene.

Pathogen Control on the Live Animal

In any HACCP program for the primary processing of meat the state of the live animal is a major critical control point. The physiological state of the animal and internal and external microbial loading are all important determinants of the final microbiological quality of derived meats. Among these factors, the presence of faeces on animal hides, fleece or skin has long been recognized as a major source of pathogens on carcasses (Roberts 1980). This is not to suggest that other factors such as plant design, slaughter procedures and adherence to good manufacturing practices, are not also important in ensuring the production of carcasses of good hygienic quality. According to a generic HACCP for raw beef of the National Advisory Committee on Microbiological Criteria for Food, preslaughter washing has a positive effect in removing soil from animals (Anon. 1993). While some countries, such as New Zealand, have accepted the value of this process, and adopted a national policy of presenting washed animals for slaughter, the efficacy of this procedure has frequently been challenged (Roberts 1980; Biss and Hathaway 1995; Bell 1997). In spite of these reservations many agencies are targeting the hide as a major control point for the control of meat hygiene and insisting on clean animals being presented for slaughter (Ridell and Korkeala 1993; Anon. 1995; Anon. 1997; Lowman *et al.* 1997).

There is little doubt that pathogens such as *Escherichia coli* O157:H7 are spread from the hide to the carcass during slaughter. This is shown in Table 1, where prior to slaughter, live cattle were inoculated on the flank and rump, over a combined area of about 800 cm^2, with a mixture of faeces and the pathogen.

TABLE 1.
THE SPREAD OF *E. COLI* O157:H7 (log_{10}cfu/cm^2) FROM INOCULATED LIVE* CATTLE HIDES TO CARCASS AND OTHER SURFACES AFTER SLAUGHTER

Carcass	Carcass Location		Surfaces: Operatives Hands	Saws	Knives	Flares+
Left side	Hind	2.82	3.68	2.81	1.92	-0.33
	Fore	-0.38				
Right side	Hind	2.86				
	Fore	1.53				

* Live animals (n = 10)
\+ Rotating blades used to trim and dehide beef carcasses
Mean inoculum level on hides -3.62 cfu/cm^2
Data: Bolton *et al.* (1997)

The resulting contamination of the carcass, the operatives and their implements, demonstrates the ease of spread of this pathogen during slaughter. This was particularly evident in terms of manual activities in that the numbers of the pathogen on the hands of the operatives were almost identical to the numbers inoculated onto the hide (Bolton *et al.* 1997). Although the animals were inoculated on the hindquarters only, both the fore and hindquarters of the carcass were subsequently contaminated. The hindquarters were most heavily contaminated and the appearance of the pathogen on the forequarter could have resulted from its redistribution during carcass washing with cold water.

The influence of excessive amounts of faecal contamination or dung on cattle, in relation to carcass contamination, is presented in Table 2. This shows that excessively dungy cattle yield carcasses with a higher level of contamination than normal animals (Ridell and Korkeala 1993).

TABLE 2.
EFFECT OF EXCESSIVE DUNG ON CATTLE HIDES ON CARCASS TOTAL COUNTS (log_{10}cfu/cm^2)

Carcass Site	Control	Excessively Dungy
Shoulder	2.14[a]	2.89[b]
Brisket	3.82[c]	4.50[d]

Different superscripts within a row or column significantly different (P<.01)
Data: Ridell and Korkeala (1993)

The data in Table 3 shows that while the numbers of excessively dungy animals being presented at a meat plant were a small percentage of the total (2.17%), good farm management practices had significantly reduced the numbers over a period of seven years (Ridell and Korkeala 1993). Most of the dungy cattle were produced during the winter months and the factory adopted a policy for handling dungy cattle. Cleaner animals were slaughtered first while dungy cattle were retained and slaughtered separately at the end of the kill. During this period line speed is slower, so that greater care can be taken with these dirty animals and the added costs for this procedure are passed onto the farmer. It is interesting to note that even with greater care being taken the dungy animals still produced carcasses with higher counts (Table 2). Regulations similar to these in Finland for grading cattle for the amount of dung on the hide have been introduced into Irish export meat plants (Anon. 1997) and in the United Kingdom (Lowman *et al.* 1997).

TABLE 3.
NUMBER AND PERCENTAGE OF DUNGY CATTLE ARRIVING AT A SLAUGHTER HOUSE IN FINLAND

Year	Number Slaughtered	Excessively Dungy	
		No.	%
1983	76,840	1670	2.17
1986	63,970	604	0.94
1990	63,711	201	0.32

Data: Ridell and Korkeala (1993)

Recognition of the equivalent problem in sheep in controlling contamination of the fleece has resulted in shearing the fleece and then washing, or washing without shearing (Biss and Hathaway 1995). When animals with a long fleece (6 cm or more) were washed with cold water, significant increases in the levels of carcass contamination were observed (Table 4). These data suggest that washing the live animal does not enhance the microbial status of the carcass, even on shorn animals. While washing did not reduce the numbers of bacteria on carcasses, other contamination, such as faecal staining, can be significantly reduced (Biss and Hathaway 1995). At the present time equipment for dagging sheep and removing faecal clods from cattle hides are being developed at CSIRO in Australia (Stapleton 1997).

Finally, in relation to live animal decontamination, dehairing cattle or defleecing sheep has been attempted in the past (Schnell *et al.* 1995; Leach 1971). The data in Table 5 shows that these approaches have not been successful. Bacterial counts were not affected by either process, although the visual appearance of the meat was improved as a result of less hairs on the carcass and on the resulting meat. The removal of the fleece and hair in these studies was very different. For the fleece, the shedding agent used (cyclophosphamide) was a drug, administered orally to the animals, while the cattle were dehaired with a chemical, sodium sulphide, applied topically. While oral defleecing avoided the pollution problems associated with dehairing, it had the disadvantage of being toxic in large doses (Dolnick *et al.* 1970). Although chemical dehairing of the live animal has not proved successful, it may be that, combined with other decontamination processes for carcasses, to be discussed below, it could have a future.

TABLE 4.
THE EFFECT OF PRE-SLAUGHTER STATUS ON LAMB CARCASS CONTAMINATION LEVELS ($log_{10}cfu/cm^2$) AFTER PELT REMOVAL

	Preslaughter Status			
	Clean Shorn	Dirty Shorn	Clean Woolly	Dirty Woolly
Washed	4.16	4.33	4.47	4.63
Unwashed	3.93	4.26	3.94	4.30
Effect of washing	N.S.	N.S.	P<.001	P<.001

Data: Biss and Hathaway, (1995)
NS = non significant

TABLE 5.
EFFECT OF CHEMICAL DEHAIRING OF BEEF OR DEFLEECING OF SHEEP ON MEAN BACTERIAL COUNTS ON CARCASSES

	Cattle ($log_{10}cfu/cm^2$)		
Treatment	Total Counts	Coliforms	*E. coli*
Dehaired	4.00a	1.96a	1.14a
Control	4.14a	1.64b	1.21a

Means in the same column followed by the same letter are not different (P< .05)

	Sheep ($log_{10}cfu/carcass$)		
Defleeced	6.53	-	-
Control	7.18	-	-

Data: Beef - Schnell *et al.* (1995); Lamb - Leach (1971)

The Influence of "Bung Tying" on Pathogen Control

Tying the bung (rectum) or sealing the rectum of animals during slaughter is designed to reduce the spread of faecal material from the rectum to the carcass. In recent years this process has been improved by tying the bung and covering with a plastic bag. The effectiveness of this additional precaution in reducing contamination on pig carcasses has been demonstrated by Nesbakken *et al.* (1994). They showed that in commercial trials the occurrence of *Yersinia enterocolitica* 0:3 on pig carcasses was significantly reduced (Table 6). When this system was introduced into commercial production in Norway in 1994 the incidence of yersiniosis in the population decreased by 25% in the following year.

TABLE 6.
EFFECT OF A PLASTIC BAG TO SEAL THE RECTUM OF PIGS ON THE OCCURRENCE OF *YERSINIA ENTEROCOLITICA* 0:3 ON PIG CARCASSES DURING SLAUGHTER

	Country			
	Norway		Sweden	
Slaughter rate (no./h)	90.0		240.0	
Bung (1) covered with plastic bag (2) uncovered	(1)	(2)	(1)	(2)
Number of *Yersinia*-positive pigs	0	7(11.7)*	1.0(1.7)	5.0(8.3)*
Differences covered vs uncovered	P<.01			
Countries	N.S.			

*Percentage
NS = not significant
Data: Nesbakken *et al.* (1994)

A system to completely automate sealing the rectum of cattle has been developed in Australia and is presently commercially available (Leemon 1997). This 'safe seal' system has undergone commercial trials and has been shown to give significantly lower levels of carcass contamination, compared to the manual system (Fig. 1).

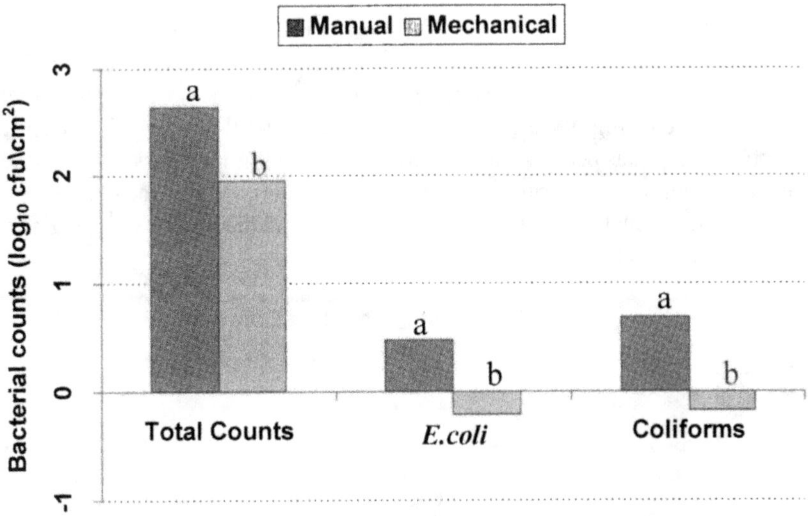

***AUSTRALIAN MEAT TECHNOLOGY SAFESEAL SYSTEM**
Data: Leemon (1997)
[ab]Means with different superscripts are significantly different ($P < 0.01$)

FIG. 1. COMPARISON BETWEEN A MANUAL AND A MECHANICAL SYSTEM TO SEAL THE BUNG OF CATTLE DURING SLAUGHTER

Trimming and Steam-Vacuuming

In order to comply with the zero tolerance criteria laid down by the US Food Safety Inspection Service (FSIS), carcasses must be free from all faecal staining prior to final washing (Anon. 1995). Trimming is an on-line process used to remove fat, small faecal spots and smears from beef carcasses. An alternative to trimming for the removal of small faecal stains is the use of steam-vacuuming. The processes of trimming and steam-vacuuming were applied to beef carcasses prior to evisceration and their ability to reduce bacterial numbers and faecal staining was assessed (Fig. 2). Steam-vacuuming was as successful in reducing bacterial numbers, including coliforms, as knife-trimming and both processes gave significant reductions compared to controls (Kochevar *et al.* 1997). Both treatments were also equally successful in removing visible faecal contamination. An added advantage of steam-vacuuming is the avoidance of producing contaminated waste meat.

Preevisceration Washing

Many HACCP systems recommend preevisceration washing or sanitizing immediately after dehiding as a means of reducing bacterial counts on the carcass at final dressing (Anon. 1993). It is carried out immediately after hide removal in order to obtain maximum effect in terms of bacterial removal. This is demonstrated in Fig. 3 which shows the added effectiveness of the preevisceration wash in reducing bacterial contamination after final washing. The basis of this improvement has been explained by Dickson (1995). If carcasses are washed soon after dehiding the ability of bacteria to adhere to the meat surface is reduced. This reduction results from a lowering of the meat surface tension which prevents bacterial adhesion.

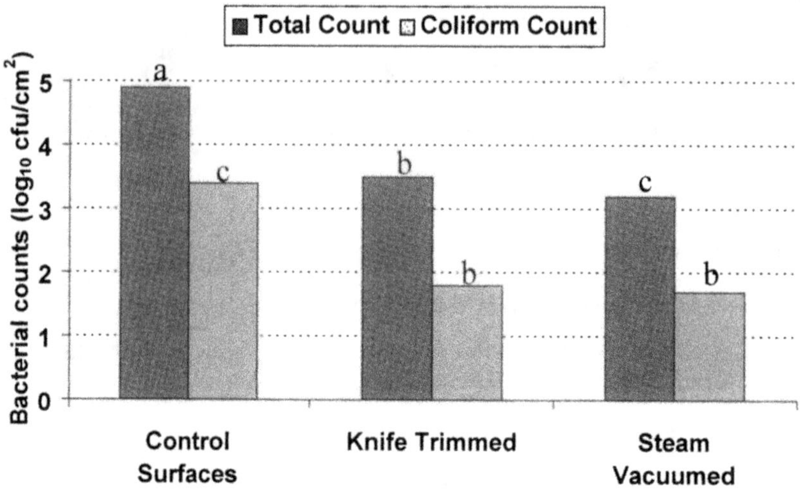

Data: Kochevar *et al.* (1997)

[abc] Means with different superscripts are significantly different ($P<0.05$)

FIG. 2. EFFECT OF STEAM VACUUMING OR KNIFE TRIMMING ON MEAN TOTAL AND COLIFORM COUNTS ($\log_{10}$ cfu/cm^2) ON BEEF CARCASSES SLAUGHTERED IN A COMMERCIAL ABATTOIR

Evisceration

Evisceration may have an adverse effect on the contamination of meat. The influence of evisceration on the *Enterobacteriaceae* counts on lamb carcasses during slaughter is shown in Fig. 4. These data were the means from four different commercial plants in Ireland and show that contamination of the sternum/abdominal area of the carcass was significantly increased as a result of evisceration (Sierra *et al.* 1997). Increased *Enterobacteriaceae* counts after evisceration may have potential as an indicator of a deterioration in sheep slaughter practices.

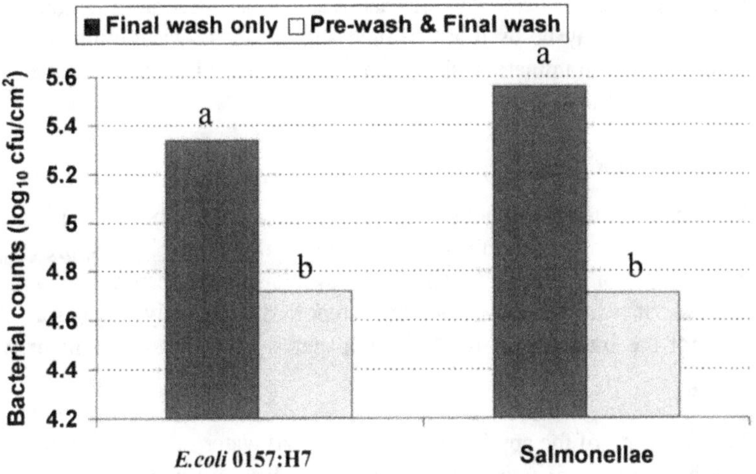

Data: Dickson (1995)

[ab] Means with different superscript letters are significantly different ($P<0.05$)

FIG. 3. EFFECT OF PRE-EVISCERATION WASHING ON BEEF CARCASSES INOCULATED WITH *E. COLI* O157:H7 OR SALMONELLAE

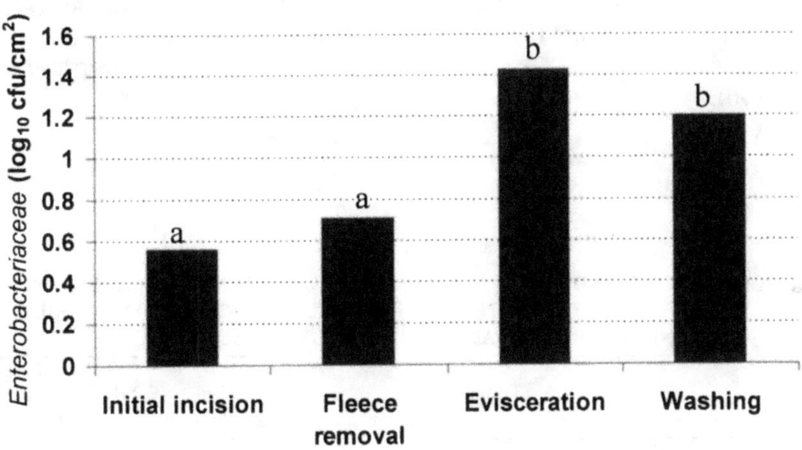

Data: Sierra *et al.* (1997)

[ab] Means with different superscript letters are significantly different ($P<0.01$)

FIG. 4. THE INFLUENCE OF PROCESSING ON *ENTEROBACTERIACEAE* COUNTS (log_{10} cfu/cm^2) ON LAMB CARCASSES

Where faecal spots occur on beef carcasses after evisceration-trimming or steam-vacuuming may be used as outlined above. Steam-vacuuming may also have a role in decontaminating sheep carcasses after evisceration as the areas involved are small.

Carcass Decontamination

In recent years the meat industry has expressed considerable interest in meat carcass decontamination systems and a number of these have been approved for use by FSIS (Anon. 1995). A variety of systems have been tested and the effectiveness of many of these have been reported previously (Siragusa 1996) and it is not the intention of the present paper to reconsider the majority of these.

(1) The efficiency of the application of hot or cold water in removing or killing bacteria has been examined by a number of different workers (Kelly *et al.* 1982; Dorsa *et al.* 1996). According to Reagan *et al.* (1996) cold or warm water (35C) is less effective than hot (80C+) and the effects are similar for aerobic and *E. coli* counts (Table 7). Cold water sprays rely on physical removal of bacteria, while bacterial injury or death requires the presence of heat. Hot water systems use up to 40 L of water per carcass, depending on the type of spray used, and decontamination is for 15 to 20 s. The water is filtered and recycled and losses are made up with potable water only. Recently it has been suggested that combined treatments with hot (70C) water at low pressure (20 psi), in combination with high pressure (125 psi) and warm water (30C) give the most effective treatment (Dorsa *et al.* 1996).

TABLE 7.
MEAN AEROBIC AND *E. COLI* COUNTS ($log_{10}cfu/cm^2$) FROM BEEF CARCASSES DELIBERATELY CONTAMINATED WITH FAECAL MATERIAL FROM THE HIDE AND DECONTAMINATED DURING NORMAL SLAUGHTER

	Control	Trimmed	*Washed (28-42C)	*Hot Washed (74-88C)
Aerobic count	4.20^a	2.88^c	3.24^b	2.20^d
E. coli	2.23^a	0.63^c	1.19^b	0.41^c

*Washed in on-line automated wash cabinets in a commercial abattoir
Means followed by different letters in the same row are statistically different P<.05.
Data: Reagan *et al.* (1996)

Washing beef carcasses with warm water (35C) may increase contamination levels. Figure 5 shows that washing with a hand-held hose, using a rise and fall stand, increased contamination at a number of sites on beef carcasses. These data indicate that washing redistributed the bacteria more generally over the different sites on the carcasses (McEvoy *et al.* 1997). In experiments where bacterial removal has been demonstrated with warm water, washing was carried out in cabinets, where the direction of water flow, pressure and temperature are all controlled (Reagan *et al.* 1996). Under these conditions positive reductions in cell numbers can be achieved as bacterial redistribution across the carcass is avoided.

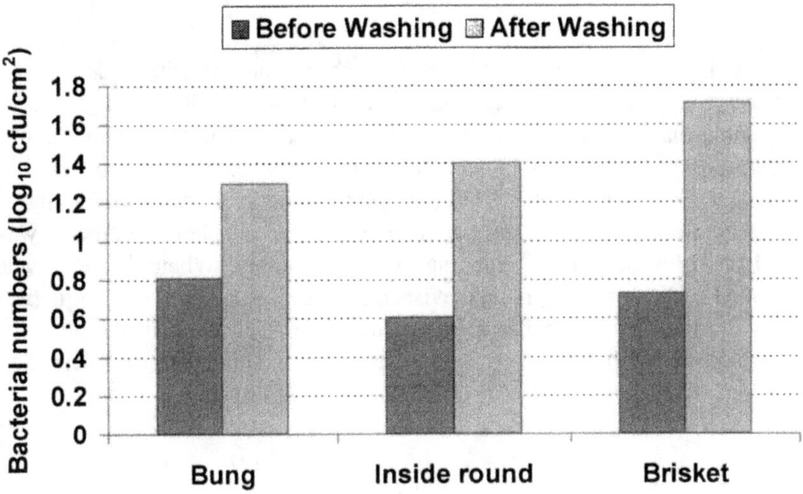

Data: McEvoy *et al.* (1997)

FIG. 5. THE EFFECT OF WASHING BEEF CARCASSES WITH WATER AT 35C ON PSYCHROTROPHIC *PSEUDOMONAS* COUNTS (log_{10} cuf/cm^2) AT DIFFERENT SITES

(2) Recently a commercial on-line decontamination system has become available using steam for short times (6 to 8 s) (Nutsch *et al.* 1997). The effectiveness of this pasteurization in reducing bacterial counts is about the same as hot water washing (Table 8). During steam pasteurization, the temperature of the surface of the carcass reaches 90-96C in about 1 s. After 6-8 s the carcass is cooled with chilled water to rapidly reduce surface temperature (Phebus *et al.* 1997).

TABLE 8.
MEAN TOTAL COUNTS ($log_{10}cfu/cm^2$) ON COMMERCIAL BEEF CARCASSES AFTER STEAM DECONTAMINATION (8 S) AND AFTER CHILLING (29 H)

Carcasses+	Control	Steam Decontaminated	Chilling
Cows	2.19[a]	0.84[b]	0.94[b]
Feedlot cattle	2.14[a]	1.03[b]	1.09[b]

Different superscripts within rows are significantly different P<01
+ Carcasses from cows and feedlot cattle, mostly steers, will have different grades
Data: Nutsch *et al.* (1997)

(3) There is a large body of evidence to show that organic acids can be successfully used to decontaminate meat (Siragusa 1996). It is generally accepted that hot acids are the most effective. Lactic acid is most commonly used and its effectiveness in decontaminating beef carcasses is illustrated in Table 9. This shows that 1% hot (55C) lactic acid applied after dehiding or evisceration at the end of the slaughter process or after both treatments was capable of significantly reducing bacterial counts. When the acid was applied both after dehiding and evisceration the reduction in contamination was significantly better than at either site alone. This confirms the previous observation on the efficacy of preevisceration washing already referred to in Fig. 3.

TABLE 9.
MEAN AEROBIC COUNTS ($log_{10}cfu/cm^2$) ON BEEF CARCASSES SPRAYED AFTER DEHIDING AND EVISCERATION WITH HOT LACTIC ACID

Sampling Time 9h	Control	Treatment With 1% Lactic Acid at 55C		
		Dehiding	Evisceration	*Both
0	3.90[a]	2.40[b]	2.20[b]	1.60[c]
72	3.50[a]	2.90[ab]	2.40[bc]	2.10[c]

* Lactic acid sprayed after dehiding and evisceration
Means with a common superscript are not significantly different P< .05
Data: Prasai *et al.* (1991)

In general, decontamination processes using either hot water, steam or hot lactic acid gave reductions in bacterial counts of about 2 logs. This reduction was generally sustained after chilling. Since hot water or steam were as effective as lactic acid or a number of other chemical decontaminating agents in removing bacteria from carcasses, it is difficult to see how they will be used by industry (Siragusa 1996). A number of chemicals, in particular chlorine or organic acids, have the major disadvantage of being highly corrosive. They also add considerable cost, particularly the acids, and environmentally would require costly systems for effective disposal.

The Effects of Line Speed on Carcass Hygiene

According to Roberts (1980) line speed may have serious implications in relation to carcass contamination. The faster the line operates the more opportunities there are for mistakes to be made and hence more contamination may occur. While this is generally true and it can be demonstrated that the effectiveness of carcass-trimming in removing contamination can be related to line speed, the precise relationship is complicated (Table 10).

TABLE 10.
THE EFFECT OF LINE SPEED ON AEROBIC COUNTS ($log_{10}cfu/cm^2$) ON BEEF CARCASSES TRIMMED UNDER COMMERCIAL CONDITIONS

	Control	Trimmed	Difference
1.	3.50	0.5	3.00
2.	4.20	2.88	1.32
1.	Carcasses stationary during trimming		
2.	Carcasses moving during normal production and trimming. (Rate: 800 - 3,200/day)		

Data: 1. Prasai *et al.* (1995)
2. Reagan *et al.* (1996)

A number of studies have investigated the effects of dressing carcasses on lines at different speeds, from very slow (160 head/day) to very fast (6000/day) (Fig. 6). Data obtained in New Zealand suggests that the mean total counts increase with line speed (Bell 1997). A study in the USA found significantly lower levels of carcass contamination at higher line speeds (Hogue *et al.* 1993). Considering the data of Hogue *et al.* (1993) the authors note a number of unexpected circumstances which may explain this anomalous situation. These include better management systems, a greater level of specialization of labor, leading to fewer cuts and the use of decontamination systems in larger establishments. Decontamination would mask many of the defects made during faster slaughter but presupposes that other plants would not use such systems, which was the case in the New Zealand work (Bell 1997).

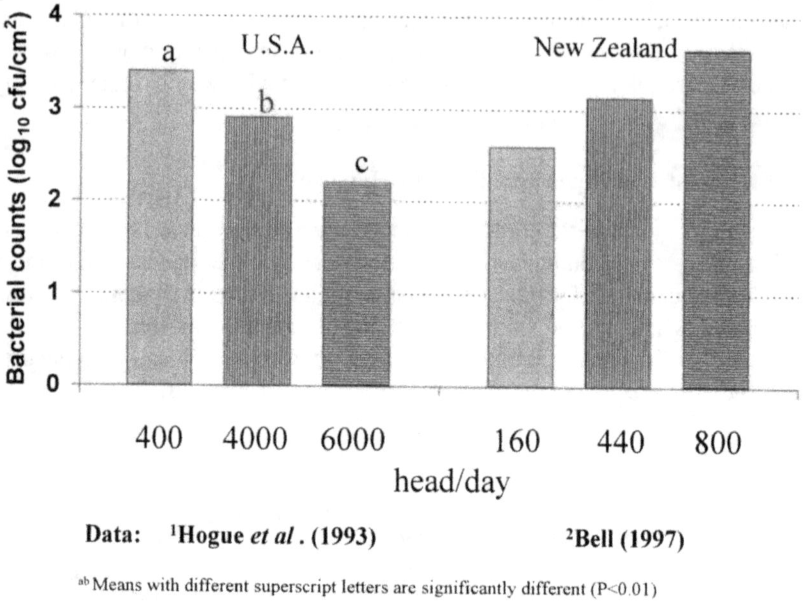

FIG. 6. TOTAL COUNTS ($\log_{10}$ cfu/cm^2) ON BEEF CARCASSES FROM CATTLE SLAUGHTER LINES OPERATING AT DIFFERENT SPEEDS

It is clear that the relationship between line speed and carcass contamination levels is not simple and is influenced by a large number of factors such as operator fatigue, knife skills, length of working day, levels of boredom and the presence/absence of proper management structures (HACCP). The most important aspect is whether or not the operatives have sufficient time to carry out their jobs. The latter is the most crucial element and is recognized in some countries where the speed of the line is regulated by the number of carcasses that an inspector can examine in an hour (Roberts 1980).

The Influence of Technology Advances on Carcass Contamination

It is often assumed that advances in technology or increased automation brings benefits in terms of carcass hygiene. Data in Table 11 broadly support this assumption, and suggests that overall reduction in the extent of carcass handling reduces contamination. In general terms, slaughter practices have developed to incorporate mechanical advances, but the changes in practices and carcass counts are not constant. In a beef plant in Australia during a 27-year period (1937-1964), no changes in bacterial numbers on carcasses were evident (Table 11); however in the succeeding 14 years, a significant improvement was noted (Grau 1979). Similar reduction in beef carcass counts have been recorded in a New Zealand plant (Keeley 1988), but in the United Kingdom modernization of a number of meat plants gave no improvements in carcass hygiene (Hudson *et al.* 1987; Whelehan *et al.* 1986).

Similar inconsistent results have been reported in relation to modernization of sheep slaughter lines in New Zealand. Keeley (1988) reported that carcass hygiene improved in one modernized plant, but not in another (Fig. 7). When two sheep plants in Ireland were examined, after an interval of 17 years, there was a significant deterioration in carcass hygiene in both (Sierra *et al.* 1997). Considerable technological changes had occurred in these plants in recent years with the installation of fleece pullers and an inverted system of carcass dressing.

TABLE 11.
INFLUENCE OF CHANGES IN SLAUGHTER TECHNOLOGY ON TOTAL COUNTS ($\log_{10}$cfu/cm^2) ON BEEF CARCASSES PROCESSED IN DIFFERENT COUNTRIES

Country	Time	Total Counts	References
	1937	3.88	Grau 1979
Australia	1964	3.90	
	1978	2.79[a]	
	1973	2.85	Keeley 1988
New Zealand	1979	2.10	
	1986	2.16	
	Original line	3.60	
	Modernized line (a)	3.57	Hudson *et al.* 1987
	(b)	3.76	
United Kingdom	Manual line	3.07	Whelehan *et al.* 1986
	Automated line	3.04	

[a]Significantly different $P<.01$)

According to Longdell (1996) and Bell and Hathaway (1996) the inverted system of lamb dressing gives improvements in bacterial numbers on carcasses. That fleece pullers can improve carcass hygiene at some sites has been shown (Field *et al.* 1991) (Table 12), but overall carcass hygiene may deteriorate as a result of faster throughputs, coupled with a deterioration in hygiene standards

(Mackey and Roberts 1993). In summary, though automation can clearly make the slaughter process less labor intensive and technologically more efficient, significant benefits in terms of carcass hygiene are not automatically achieved when such systems are introduced.

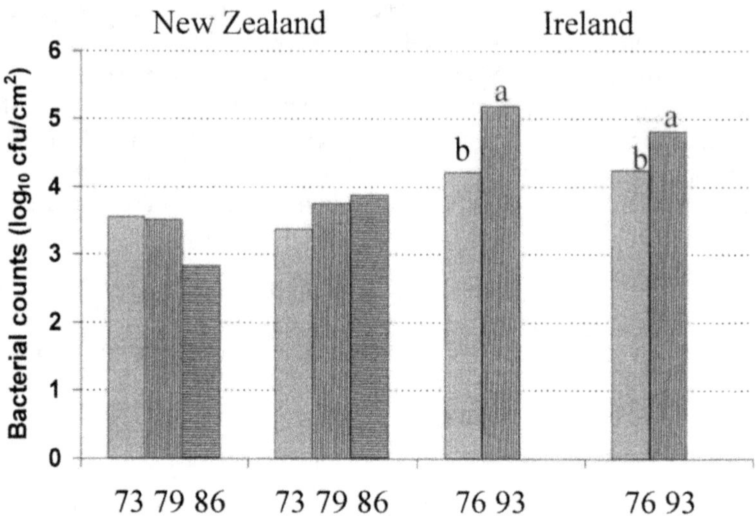

Data: **Keeley (1988)** **Sierra *et al.* (1997)**

[ab] Means with different superscript letters are significantly different ($P<0.01$)

FIG. 7. INFLUENCE OF CHANGES IN SLAUGHTER TECHNOLOGY ON TOTAL COUNTS ($\log_{10}/cm^2$) ON LAMB CARCASSES PROCESSED IN DIFFERENT COUNTRIES

TABLE 12.
THE EFFECTIVENESS OF A PELT PULLER, COMPARED TO HAND REMOVAL, IN REDUCING TOTAL COUNTS ON LAMB CARCASSES ($\log_{10}cfu/cm^2$)

	Animal Fleece			
Carcass Site	Long		Short	
	Puller	Hand	Puller	Hand
Shoulder	2.46^a	2.15^a	2.55^a	2.32^a
Leg	1.82^a	2.31^b	1.86^a	2.32^b

Different superscripts in the same row differ ($P<.05$)
Data: Field *et al.* (1991)

CONCLUSIONS

The hide or fleece of the live animal is generally recognized as the single largest source of contamination of beef and lamb carcasses. While decontamination of the live animal presents many practical difficulties, it should be addressed as a priority in relation to pathogen control. The introduction of changes in technology or processing should be assessed in relation to their efficacy in reducing carcass contamination. These changes should be considered in relation to an overall HACCP plan and should only be accepted where there is a proven relationship between a reduction in contamination and the introduction of the new technology.

REFERENCES

ANON. 1993. Generic HACCP for raw beef. National Advisory Committee on Microbiological Criteria for Foods US Department of Agriculture. Food Microbiol. *10*, 449–488.

ANON. 1995. Pathogen reduction: hazard analysis critical control point (HACCP) systems, proposed rule. Federal Register *60*, 6773–6888.

ANON. 1997. Clean Cattle Policy. Department of Agriculture, Food and Forestry, Dublin.

BELL, R.G. 1997. Distribution and sources of microbial contamination on beef carcasses. J. Appl. Microbiol. *82*, 292–300.

BELL, R.G. and HATHAWAY, S.C. 1996. The hygienic efficiency of conventional and inverted lamb dressing systems. J. Appl. Microbiol. *81*, 225–234.

BISS, M.E. and HATHAWAY, S.C. 1995. Microbiological and visible contamination of lamb carcasses according to pre-slaughter presentation status: implications for HACCP. J. Food Prot. *58* (7), 7776–783.

BOLTON, D.J., BYRNE, C. and SHERIDAN, J.J. 1997. The transfer of *Escherichia coli* O157:H7 from the contaminated hide to the carcass during routine slaughter. Unpublished data. The National Food Centre, Dublin.

DICKSON, J.S. 1995. Susceptibility of pre-evisceration washed beef carcasses to contamination by *Escherichia coli O157:H7* and Salmonellae. J. Food Prot. *58*, 1065–1068.

DOLNICK, E.H., LINDAHL, I.L., REYNOLDS, P., TERRILL, C.E. and DICKINSON, H.L. 1970. CPA lethality in sheep at high dose levels. J. Anim. Sci. *31*, 220.

DORSA, W.J., CUTTER, C.N. and SIRAGUSA, G.R. 1996. Effectiveness of a steam-vacuum sanitizer for reducing *Escherichia coli* O157:H7 inoculated to beef carcass surface tissue. Lett. Appl. Microbiol. *23*, 61–63.

FIELD, R.A., KALCHAYANAND, N., ROZBEH, M. and ANDERSEN, M.K. 1991. Influence of a pelt puller on microbiological quality of lamb. Proc. West. Sec., Amer. Soc. Anim. Sci. *42*, 147–148.

GRAU, F. 1979. Fresh meats: bacterial association. Arch. Lebensmittelhyg. *30*, 87–91.

HOGUE, A.T. *et al.* 1993. Bacterial on beef briskets and ground beef: correlation with slaughter volume and ante-mortem condemnation. J. Food Prot. *56*, 110–113, 119.

HUDSON, W.R., ROBERTS, T.A. and WHELEHAN, O.P. 1987. Bacteriological status of beef carcasses at a commercial abattoir before and after slaughterline improvements. Epidem. Inf. *98*, 81–86.

KEELEY, G.M. 1988. The microbiological status of meat from some typical New Zealand meat slaughtering and processing lines. Proc. 34th Internat. Cong. of Meat Sci. and Tech., pp. 504–507, Brisbane, Australia.

KELLY, C.A., LYNCH, B. and McLOUGHLIN, A.J. 1982. The effect of spray washing on the development of bacterial numbers and storage life of lamb carcasses. J. Appl. Bact. *53*, 335–341.

KOCHEVAR, S.L., SOFOS, J.N., BOLIN, R.R., REAGAN, J.O. and SMITH, G.C. 1997. Steam vacuuming as a pre-evisceration intervention to decontaminate beef carcasses. J. Food Prot. *60*, 107–113.

LEACH, T.M. 1971. Preliminary observations on the chemical de-fleecing of sheep as a means of reducing carcass contamination. Proc. Eur. Meet. Meat Res. Workers, pp. 161–166, Bristol.

LEEMON, H. 1997. Australian Meat Technology Safe Seal System 500. Unpublished data. Australian Meat Technology Pty Ltd., 1820 Ipswich Road, Rocklea, Queensland, Australia.

LONGDELL, G.R. 1996. Recent developments in sheep and beef processing in Australia. Meat Sci. *43*, 165–174.

LOWMAN, B.G., SYNGE, B. and CALDOW, G. 1997. Producing clean slaughter cattle. Technical Note, T468 SAC, West Mains Road, Edinburgh, EH9 3JG.

MACKEY, B.M. and ROBERTS, T.A. 1993. Improving slaughter hygiene using HACCP and monitoring. Fleischwirtschaft *73*, 58–61.

McEVOY, J., SHERIDAN, J.J. and McGUIRE, L. 1997. The effect of cold water washing on beef carcass contamination. Unpublished data. The National Food Centre, Dublin.

NESBAKKEN, T., NERBRINK, E., RØTTERUD, O.J. and BORCH, E. 1994. Reduction of *Yersinia enterocolitica* and *Listeria* spp. on pig carcasses by enclosure of the rectum during slaughter. Int. J. Food Microbiol. *23*, 197–208.

NUTSCH, A.L *et al.* 1997. Evaluation of a steam pasteurisation process in a commercial beef processing facility. J. Food Prot. *60*, 485–492.

PHEBUS, R.K. *et al.* 1997. Comparison of steam pasteurisation and other methods for reduction of pathogens on surfaces of freshly slaughtered beef. J. Food Prot. *60,* 476–484.

PRASAI, R.K., ACUFF, G.R., LUCIA, L.M., HALE, D.S., SAVELL, J.W. and MORGAN, J.B. 1991. Microbiological effects of acid decontamination of beef carcasses at various locations in processing. J. Food Prot. *54,* 868–872.

PRASAI, R.K., PHEBUS, R.K., GARCIA ZEPEDA, C.M., KASTNER, C.L., BOYLE, A.E. and FUNG, D.Y.C. 1995. Effectiveness of trimming and/or washing on microbiological quality of beef carcasses. J. Food Prot. *58,* 1114–1117.

REAGAN, J.O. *et al.* 1996. Trimming and washing of beef carcasses as a method of improving the microbiological quality of meat. J. Food Prot. *59,* 751–756.

RIDELL, J. and KORKEALA, H. 1993. Special treatment during slaughtering in Finland of cattle carrying an excessive load of dung: meat hygienic aspects. Meat Sci. *35*, 223–228.

ROBERTS, T.A. 1980. Contamination of meat: the effects of slaughter practices on the bacteriology of the red meat carcass. Royal Soc. Health *100*, 3–9.

SIERRA, M.L., SHERIDAN, J.J. and McGUIRE, L. 1997. Microbial quality of lamb carcasses during processing and the acridine orange direct count technique (a modified DEFT) for rapid enumeration of total viable counts. Int. J. Food Microbiol. *36*, 61–67.

SIRAGUSA, G.R. 1996. The effectiveness of carcass decontamination systems for controlling the presence of pathogens on the surface of meat animal carcasses. In *HACCP: An Integrated Approach to Assuring the Microbiological Safety of Meat and Poultry*. (J.J. Sheridan, R.L. Buchanan and T.J. Montville, eds.) pp. 89–98, Food & Nutrition Press, Trumbull, CT.

SCHNELL, T.D. *et al.* 1995. Effects of post-exsanguination dehairing on the microbial load and visual cleanliness of beef carcasses. J. Food Prot. *58,* 1297–1302.

STAPLETON, P. 1997. Beef and sheep carcass decontamination equipment for the removal of faecal clods and dags from beef and sheep. Personal communication. CSIRO, Brisbane Laboratory, Cannon Hill, Queensland, Australia.

WHELEHAN, O.P., HUDSON, W.R. and ROBERTS, T.A. 1986. Microbiology of beef carcasses before and after slaughterline automation. J. Hyg. Camb. *96*, 205–216.

CHAPTER 12

RESIDUE TESTING AND CONTROL STRATEGIES

JAMES D. MACNEIL

Centre for Veterinary Drug Residues
Canadian Food Inspection Agency
Saskatoon, Saskatchewan, Canada S7N 2R3

ABSTRACT

The need for residue testing and controls basically derives from two imperatives, the safety of the food supply and requirements imposed in trade. Maximum residue limits (MRLs) for pesticides, veterinary drugs, intentional food additives and potential contaminants, such as mycotoxins, are set for various food commodities based on toxicological assessment. Regulatory testing on domestically produced goods reveals the prevalence of a particular residue in a specific food commodity and also serves as a means to assess the effectiveness of the product registration system, while testing conducted on imports is primarily a verification of the effectiveness of the regulatory program in the exporting country. For industry, testing is required to demonstrate due diligence or to ensure that a product meets the specifications of an export market or a specific contract. Testing programs should be appropriate to meet the intended use. A survey to determine incidence of violations requires a test that detects residues above the MRL, while a dietary exposure study requires methodology that detects residues with the maximum achievable sensitivity. Tests conducted to certify a product for export or to fulfill the requirements of a contract should ensure that the product is in compliance with the market or contract requirement. If the requirement is "no detectable residues", a very sensitive test method may be required. In many countries, there is a developing consensus that while government has a role in conducting work that is in the public interest, such as ensuring the safety of the food supply within a level of statistical assurance, it is ultimately the producer of the food who is responsible for the safety of the product or for ensuring that the product meets market or contract requirements. Various aspects of this changing regulatory, trade and consumer environment will be considered, with examples of the roles now played by governments and industry to ensure the safety and quality of food products.

INTRODUCTION

The world in which we live has undergone major and rapid changes in the past fifty years. We have emerged from a postwar era in the late 1940's, when the availability of sufficient food was a major concern for many people in Europe and Asia, through a period of changing diets, with increasing exposure to foods from other countries and cultures, to the present time, where much of the food we eat is produced in distant parts of the world. This has led to an increased international emphasis on standardization of quality and sanitary requirements, in part because the increased use of crop protection chemicals and veterinary drug products in modern agriculture has required increased regulatory intervention. In addition, the consuming public is more aware of and concerned about potential residues, be they chemical or microbiological, in their food. With this growing need for assurance not only of the security, but also of the safety, of our food supply has come also the awareness that government regulators are not the only ones responsible for ensuring that this need is met. The role of producers, manufacturers, retailers and consumers must also be considered in this equation.

Residue testing and control programs are derived from two fundamental considerations, consumer concerns regarding the safety of the food supply and requirements imposed in trade. The two are not exclusive, but rather are closely linked. Regulatory standards in each country reflect, to some extent, the awareness of the issues and the acceptance of particular practices by the consumers in that country. Thus, we see situations occur at the international level where a practice that is commonly accepted in one country may, for historical, cultural or other reasons, be banned in another. International organizations such as the Codex Alimentarius (jointly established in 1962 by the Food and Agriculture Organization of the United Nations and the World Health Organization) provide a forum for discussion and consensus building, but also by their nature must rely on sound science, rather than opinion, in their decision-making. The standards developed by Codex Committees must therefore be based on the best available scientific information and accepted evaluation practices. The process must also be transparent and readily understood.

Maximum residue limits (MRLs) set through the Codex Alimentarius are based on the same assessment principles used by European Union, North American and other national regulatory authorities, and with the intention of providing a harmonized international standard. However, this does not mean that the final MRL (for residues of a compound in a commodity) that is adopted as a Codex standard is necessarily the same in all countries. International trade agreements attempt to reduce barriers created in such situations by referencing Codex standards but, in the meantime, it is usually the exporter who will suffer the consequences when a product is rejected at import due to differences in

MRLs or other regulated requirements. There is also a growing market for "residue-free" products, or for products certified to meet a stricter residue standard than has been imposed by a regulatory authority. These requirements will normally be established by individual supplier contracts and may not involve national regulatory authorities. Thus, residue testing is required not only to ensure that foods meet a standard for safety set by a national authority, but also to meet specific market requirements. Tests conducted to meet the first of these requirements will not necessarily also satisfy the second requirement.

REQUIREMENTS FOR A REGULATORY PROGRAM

The Codex Alimentarius Volume 3, *Residues of Veterinary Drugs in Foods*, outlines some general principles on which an effective residue control program can be based (FAO 1993). These include:

(1) establishment of a regulatory authority responsible for inspection and laboratory analyses;
(2) establishment of an inspection program, including residue controls and authority to deal with residues not in compliance with MRLs;
(3) establishment of a registry of approved products;
(4) regulation of the manufacture, distribution, sale and use of approved products;
(5) establishment of procedures for safety and efficacy assessment of the products and the safety of residues which may occur in foods;
(6) establishment of sampling procedures for food products, including the identification of residues which pose the greatest health risk (risk management), identifying numbers of samples to be collected, the statistical basis and the particular food commodity and amount to be sampled;
(7) identification of testing methods to be used;
(8) development of a quality assurance program for laboratory tests;
(9) development of an educational program.

The above list is not considered to contain the only requirements, but rather to constitute a minimum set of criteria to which individual countries may add other specific items to meet local or national conditions. While these principles have been referenced for the regulation of veterinary drug residues, most could also be considered applicable for the regulation of pesticides or food additives and also for dealing with potential contaminants.

In general terms, regulatory testing on domestically produced goods provides an assessment of the prevalence of a particular residue in a specific food commodity produced within the country and also serves as a means to assess the effectiveness of the product registration system, while testing conducted on imports is primarily a verification of the effectiveness of the regulatory program in the exporting country (FAO 1993). The usual basis for a survey program, when there is no reason to suspect a high rate of non-compliance, is to test sufficient samples to detect a 1% incidence of residues above the maximum residue limit (MRL) with 95% confidence. In a given population, such as a "national herd", this requires a random collection of 299 samples within a defined period. For a national monitoring program, this is usually taken to be over a year, or the portion of the year that reflects a production period. Based on such survey results, subsequent surveillance testing may be undertaken and then the frequency of sampling is usually related to the past history of compliance, whether in dealing with domestic or imported products.

For testing programs where the objective is to determine compliance with an MRL, the tests used are either rapid qualitative tests designed to detect samples that exceed the MRL or quantitative laboratory tests that have been validated with a limit of quantitation at one-half the MRL (or lower). In addition, national authorities may conduct total dietary exposure, or market basket surveys, designed to assess the exposure of a typical consumer to various residues which may be present in foods. For such surveys, where the objective is to detect any exposure to residues, analytical tests may be applied which are much more sensitive than those used to determine compliance with an MRL.

It is necessary to digress for a moment to consider some definitions and their impact on this issue. Compounds which may result in the presence of residues in foods are assessed on the basis of their potential toxic effects to consumers. The term "acceptable daily intake", or "ADI", is used to designate the amount of a substance that the average individual can safely consume every day of their lives, without suffering any adverse effect. This assessment often includes a safety factor of 10 or greater to allow for differences within the population, differences between humans and the animal species in which toxic effects were demonstrated, or other such factors. The ADI, therefore, is the result of a risk assessment. From the ADI, Maximum Residue Limits (MRLs) are set for specific commodities and an estimate, based on a standard food basket, is made of the potential maximum daily intake of the residue if all foods in which the residue could appear were consumed. This "theoretical maximum daily intake" should not exceed the ADI. Furthermore, when agricultural chemicals or food additives are used as approved by regulatory authorities, such use should not result in residues which exceed the MRL. The purpose of the typical national survey program is to ensure that residues in excess of the MRLs occur with a low frequency, so that the risk of any one individual consuming foods that would cause them to ingest the ADI every day is very low. This is not to say that a particular cut of meat, a vegetable or a piece of fruit that we eat at a given meal will be free of residues, or free of residues below the MRL. Rather, it means that exposure to residues above an MRL should be unusual and infrequent. Establishment of an MRL is therefore a part of risk management.

For many people, basing the prevalence of a particular residue in the food supply on the analysis of 299 samples may not give great confidence as to the residue status of the food on the dinner table. In addition, for some consumers, the possibility that residues are present in foods at detectable levels below an MRL may not be sufficient. They want a higher level of assurance, or less risk of exposure, and this is where the crossover from a national issue of food safety to an individual concern occurs. This is where we begin to face the issue of whose responsibility is the safety of that product. In general terms, it is accepted that government has a major role to play in the public interest to ensure that food is produced within a regulatory structure that protects the individual consumer from a diet of contaminated products.

Realistically, however, every single product cannot be checked for all the potential residues which might be present. Instead, we must rely on a statistical sampling to give us a picture of the residues which may be present in the food. The role of government regulatory authorities, therefore, is understood today in many countries as the setting of standards and then auditing to ensure that these standards are generally met. While the average consumer is considered to be protected from undue risk by national survey programs and the regulatory actions which may result, an individual consumer still may unknowingly be exposed to some residues in some of the foods they will consume throughout their lives. The more infrequent individual consumers wish such potential exposure to be, the more this will add to the cost of production, simply because increasing the probability that the food contains no residues above the MRL may require more conservative use of agricultural chemicals, such as longer withdrawal periods from treatment to harvest supported by more testing to provide a higher degree of confidence in a lower targeted rate of non-compliance. Such changes in agricultural practices are not only potentially more expensive, but in some cases counter-productive in terms of efficacy of the treatment. Analytical tests are expensive, so more tests conducted by industry or government add to the production cost. As an example, while a 1% rate of non-compliance may be detected in a population with 95% confidence by testing 299 random samples, the detection of a 0.1% rate of non-compliance with 99% confidence requires the analysis of 4603 random samples. The detection of a lower rate of non-compliance (i.e., <0.1%) or increasing the confidence level to 99.9% or higher proportionally increases the number of tests that are required.

Increasingly, therefore, responsibility for the safety and quality of individual products or lots is evolving to the industry, with the consumer having a role in deciding at purchase on the acceptability of each product. Consumers who wish to use food products that, whenever possible, are certified as "residue-free" must realize that the production and certification of such goods may, as noted above, entail additional costs for the production and certification. For the majority of consumers, however, who purchase the food items that are produced under typical national regulatory systems which require compliance with MRLs, there remains the issue that the individual consumer who does not like the look, feel, smell or condition of a food product, should not only refuse to buy it, but should also speak to the retailer about the acceptability of the product. In a competitive marketplace, there should be a penalty for poor service. While this is fine in theory, the question remains as to whether it works, with each sector — government, industry, consumer — accepting a share of responsibility for food safety and quality.

TEST KITS AND RESIDUE CONTROL

A key element in many residue detection programs, whether used as part of a regulatory program by government inspectors or in an industry-based quality program, is the availability of suitable rapid tests. Successful introduction of such tests to supplement or replace laboratory testing requires a rapid test that has been validated for the intended purpose. A test that has been developed and validated for the detection of penicillin in fluid milk, for example, is not necessarily suitable for the determination of penicillin in yogurt or in beef liver. The test must be shown experimentally to be applicable to each type of sample matrix to which it is to be applied. A sample matrix, put simply, is the particular sample material to be tested, such as beef liver, whole carrots or tomato juice. Experiments which must be conducted include the determination of the test sensitivity for the residue in the target sample matrix, the interferences that may occur, the rate of false positive results and the repeatability. Protocols have been described which can be used for such evaluations (AOAC 1991) and, for some applications, test kits are available which have received third party certification for specific applications.

The availability of such a test, applied within a regulatory program, can have a significant effect in the reduction of the rate of non-compliance for a targeted residue, as it permits a much higher rate of random sampling, with the result that a much lower rate of non-compliance can be detected with a high degree of confidence than can be achieved with the typical 299 sample survey. The introduction of such screening tests also permits the reallocation of laboratory resources to the confirmation of suspected positive samples, instead of the analysis of survey samples which are predominantly in compliance with the MRL. An example which illustrates this is the evolution of the residue control programs for sulphonamides in pork in the United States and Canada.

Typically, sulphamethazine is included in grower rations to protect hogs from gastrointestinal infections; however, sulphamethazine should not be included in finisher rations, so there usually is a requirement that a non-medicated ration be fed for a minimum of 14 days prior to slaughter. The introduction of residue surveys to determine non-compliance revealed that violation rates as high as 13.1% were observed in the United States in 1977 (Van Houweling 1981), while a violation rate of 9.9% was reported in Canada for 1979/80 (Neidert *et al.* 1985). Until the early 1990's, residue control programs in Canada were based on analysis of the 299 sample random survey described earlier. Combined with a pre-test program for farms identified as having produced hogs with residues at violative levels, a feed-testing program and an education program for the industry, the violation rate was reduced to about 1% by 1990 (Food Inspection Directorate 1990). Following the development of the Sulfa-On-Site (SOS) Test by the United States Department of Agriculture and the introduction of this test at slaughter plants in the United States and Canada, testing frequency increased dramatically. In the 1995/96 fiscal year, for example, over 58,000 hogs were tested at Canadian slaughter plants using the SOS test, with a compliance rate of 99.79% (Food Inspection Directorate 1996). In addition, it was observed that repeat violations had become very rare.

This illustrates the effectiveness of a test applied at an appropriate point in the system to achieve the desired result. In the case of sulphonamides, or other medicating ingredients normally supplied on a herd basis in feed or water, testing after slaughter is certainly a useful means to determine a noncompliance rate; however, it is not necessarily the most effective way to eliminate the problem. Testing at the point of slaughter, or preferably before, to ensure that the lot of animals is in compliance has obvious advantages for all parties. Firstly, and most importantly, it greatly reduces the risk of consumer exposure to unwanted residues. Secondly, it eliminates problems at the slaughter plant, such as occur when lots are detained pending further testing. Finally, it saves the producer from an unnecessary financial loss and possible legal sanctions.

RESIDUE CONTROL AND HACCP

In many countries, there is a developing view that while government has a role in conducting work that is in the public interest, such as ensuring the safety of the food supply within a level of statistical assurance, it is ultimately the producer of the food who is responsible for the safety of the product or for ensuring that the product meets market or contract requirements. Thus, while in some countries we now see less regulatory testing by government agencies for some residues, we see increased involvement in testing by companies or producer groups in response to market opportunities, potential liabilities or as part of a quality system based on the principles of Hazard Analysis and Critical Control Points (HACCP). The introduction of a HACCP system is seen by some knowledgeable individuals as resulting in an increased demand for laboratory testing, not less, with resulting benefits for food-testing laboratories (Clapp 1997).

Some concepts used in the applications of HACCP to the control of microbiological residues in foods may also be applicable to the control of chemical residues. For example, in the dairy industry, one of the highly regulated agri-food sectors, it is common for each dairy to impose a testing regimen on each of the producers with which it deals to reduce the risk of chemical residues in the product received for manufacture. In North America, the dairy-testing program for veterinary drug residues is under the supervision of government agencies, but most of the actual testing is conducted by the dairies themselves. The ability to establish such a residue control program is predicated on the availability of simple and inexpensive rapid tests which provide a positive/negative indication of the residue status of the product. Typically, each tanker load of milk is tested for antimicrobial residues and any lot that tests positive as a potential violation is discarded. This approach is taken both to protect the very high reputation for safety and quality of milk products, as well for the equally serious concern that no residues are present which could interfere in the production of cultured products, such as cheese and yogurt.

If we think back for a moment to our statistical sampling model, it becomes evident that the use of such rapid tests is the key to increasing the frequency of testing and, therefore, the statistical confidence in the detection of samples not in compliance. Where samples can be taken which are representative of a bulk lot of a product, whether milk from a milk tanker or animals randomly selected from a herd or apples from an orchard, those random samples should reflect the residue status of the remainder of the product, provided that all have been exposed to the same regimen.

When we apply the concepts of HACCP to residue control, we must first recognize that the registration process for a veterinary drug is, in itself, consistent with a HACCP approach, as it attempts to set out set of conditions for use which provide the necessary treatment for the animal while minimizing the risk of resultant residues. As stated earlier, the effectiveness of this process can be audited, at least in part, through the results of a statistical testing of the national herd for residues; however, there are still elements in the system that though accident or deliberate misuse, could result in residues in the food products from treated animals. Taking a HACCP approach, in the case of sulphamethazine residues in swine discussed previously, we would identify the major potential sources of residues as feed contamination and poor sanitary practices. Regular cleaning of the pens, combined with testing of the feed and changeover to nonmedicated feed at the appropriate time, should ensure that animals presented for slaughter are in compliance. If the industry recognizes the value of this approach, both in eliminating costly detention of product and, more importantly, as a marketing tool, then the answer seems clear. It is in the interest of the producers and the slaughter plants to institute a residue control program, with the appropriate tests applied at the right points in the system, usually before the lot leaves the farm, or certainly prior to slaughter. In the case of sulphamethazine, such a system would include testing of the feed at regular intervals and random testing of urine or other fluid from animals randomly selected from within the herd to ensure that unwanted residues are not present. For other medicating ingredients, an evaluation would be required to identify the necessary control points, including that the appropriate quantity of the ingredient was included in the feed or water, that no cross-contamination occurred and that the appropriate withdrawal period was observed. Appropriate check points might include testing of the feed, record-keeping or live animal testing, depending on the compound used, its persistence, distribution and potential for cross-contamination.

If producers and slaughter plants adopt this approach, then the regulatory agency should be able to reduce its involvement in testing to that required to provide a statistical assurance of a desired level of compliance. The current approach of government inspectors using the SOS or other tests to monitor for compliance at the slaughter plants has certainly been demonstrated as an effective means of reducing the incidence of residue violations, but it could be argued that the result is due to the financial penalties associated with detaining or condemning of carcasses. If HACCP principles were adopted by the producers, there should be virtually no violations, other than the truly accidental ones, to detect.

A logical question might therefore be why we have not instituted such programs to control all residues. The main reason is that it is not quite as simple as it appears on the surface. If we are to predict the possibility of residues in tissues at slaughter based on a test conducted on a blood or urine sample, we have to know the distribution and depletion profile of the compound in that fluid relative to the edible tissues. In some cases, such as sulphamethazine in swine, this is known, but for some other drugs or other food animal species, the information has not been generated or is not readily available. Also, there are some drugs which will persist in certain tissues long after they are non-detectable in body fluids, so such a test strategy is not universally applicable.

Some interesting developments may be observed in the relationships between government regulatory agencies, producer groups and the veterinary drug industry, where interests coincide, as in residue prevention. Several collaborative projects are currently underway in my laboratory and these are, I believe, typical of the cooperation that should occur. One study relates to our national testing program for sulphonamide residues in pigs. When one or more animals from a lot test positive for sulphonamide residues at slaughter, it has been a common practice to detain the entire lot pending testing in a government laboratory of liver and muscle samples from no more than five of the carcasses. If any of the muscle samples are found to exceed the MRL, then the remaining carcasses are either detained until tested at the producer's expense or are condemned. At a test cost of $60 or more per sample, this option has not been particularly attractive for producers. In cooperation with the Canadian Pork Council and a test kit manufacturer, research has been conducted to determine if a test developed for sulphonamide residues in milk could be adapted to test pork muscle. With some refinements to the extraction procedure, we have been able to adapt the kit and test it in several slaughter plants. The modifications were successful and negotiations are now underway to have the test accepted by our Agency. If accepted, the result will be that the industry will have available a rapid test that can be used at the slaughter plant to clear or reject suspect carcasses, within a few hours and at a cost of under $5 per test.

Similar projects are underway involving our laboratory, veterinary drug manufacturers and test kit manufacturers to identify and validate rapid tests that can be used reliably by the industry to eliminate animals with other specific residues from the production system. This is a critical issue for companies with export contracts which demand a product with no detectable residue of these compounds. Detection sensitivities of the rapid test must be equivalent to, or preferably superior to, the analytical sensitivities of the tests used by the importing countries. In this situation, the problem is not one wherein the product does not comply with the requirements of the country of origin. Rather, the product must comply with an importer's more stringent requirement, be it a standard set by regulatory authorities in the importing country, or a market demand by consumers.

A single approach, however, is not applicable in all cases. While in some situations control of the medicating ingredient given in the feed or water is a "critical control point", there are other cases, particularly with the use of injectable drugs, where record-keeping by the producer, possibly combined with segregation of the treated animal, is "critical". For many agricultural chemicals, the highest risk of residues present at slaughter (or at harvest) is posed when the mandatory withdrawal time from treatment to slaughter (harvest) has not been observed. This has frequently been linked with poor record-keeping. Similarly, residues may also be linked to extra-label use, either by applying more of the product than is recommended on the label, or by applying the product in an unauthorized manner. Avoidance of residues at harvest or slaughter therefore is primarily a responsibility of the producer of the goods who has applied, or arranged for the application, of the chemical. An understanding of and compliance with the instructions for use, combined with accurate record-keeping, is therefore fundamental to residue avoidance at primary production level.

In a HACCP-based system, following the registration process, the first line of defense becomes the primary producer, who has a responsibility to ensure that agrochemicals are used as intended. The intended use is established by regulatory authorities, but it is the individual user who must take responsibility for how the product is used. Thus, approved dosage levels, mode of application and withdrawal times are all critical factors identified during the registration process for the use of a veterinary drug in a food-producing animal which, if followed, should ensure that the final product is in compliance with an established Maximum Residue Limit. The primary producer therefore must know and observe these requirements and, in the case of ubiquitous substances such as sulphamethazine, where accidental contamination has frequently occurred, prudence dictates the use of suitable rapid tests to be applied to both the feed and the animals to guard against accidental contamination. Good record-keeping ensures that the right test can be applied at the appropriate time, or that suitable withdrawal periods are applied when no rapid test is available to confirm the residue status.

The next level in the food production chain, the slaughter house or food processor, should reasonably be expected to insist on certain performance standards from those who supply them with the raw materials that they process. In addition to the application of grade standards for physical appearance, it is not unreasonable that they should also request disclosure of any treatment regimen with veterinary drugs, pesticides or other chemicals which may result in residues in foods. As an example, the international marketing organization for the pork industry in Saskatchewan, Canada, where our laboratory is located, has started a pilot study with 25 producers, varying from small family farms to large hog operations, to institute a quality system to control veterinary drug residues. Education, record-keeping, feed-testing and final product-testing all will be a part of this effort to ensure that animals presented for slaughter are free of residues which are in violation of Canadian or international standards. Similar industry initiatives are found in other parts of the world.

One can look, for example, to experience in the aquaculture industry in some jurisdictions, where all veterinary drugs are to be used by prescription only, with each prescription and use registered in a database. Fish are then pretested for the residue after observation of the mandatory withdrawal period for the treatment to ensure compliance with MRLs before the total lot is approved for slaughter.

As we move through the other links in the production chain, such as the wholesaler and retailer, it is again reasonable that they should require some assurance from their suppliers that the food provided is in compliance with regulatory standards. Thus, a supplier declaration of what agrochemicals have been used, at the producer level, with appropriate declarations of quality assurance systems at the various subsequent levels of food processing and marketing, should enable the identification of check points to ensure that the system is working. If we take the case of a producer declaration that they have observed all regulations for any chemicals that they have used, a random testing at the point of first processing of the product, be it a slaughter house for meat or a packing plant for fruit, should ensure that the producers are indeed in compliance. Responsibility for this testing should be recognized as a shared responsibility. There is an obvious public interest in ensuring that safety standards are met, so regulatory authorities must have a means of assurance that the system is working as planned; however, there is also a responsibility on the industry at its various component levels to ensure the safety and quality of the products. The more this philosophy is accepted and demonstrated through quality assurance systems, the less intrusive should the role of the government inspection system become. This is not to say, however, that government inspection should be eliminated, but rather that it should change from being "the quality system" to auditing the quality system. The statistically based government monitoring program described earlier continues to provide such an audit, but the self-monitoring approach recommended for the producers and food processors should ensure that findings of residues in excess of the MRL for products used under the conditions of registration should be an extremely unusual event.

As another example of industry-government cooperation, let us consider the recent developments in the United Kingdom (Kay 1997). Food laws require that the seller demonstrate "due diligence" by taking reasonable steps to ensure that products offered for sale are in compliance with safety standards. Within the United Kingdom, two testing programs have been conducted for veterinary drug residues. One of these is the "statutory testing program" required by the European Union, in which random samples, collected at slaughter plants by government inspectors, are tested in government-designated laboratories. The cost of the testing is covered by a per-animal charge at slaughter. In addition, there is a "non-statutory" program which includes animal-derived foods available for sale in the United Kingdom, with sample collection primarily at the retail level. Recently, an agreement has been reached between regulatory authorities and some major retailers that the retailers will cover the cost of the sample collection, according to government specifications, for many of the samples collected in the non-statutory test program. Results of tests on samples collected in each retailer's establishments are provided to the retailer for trace-back and all affected retailers are notified of any samples from a common supplier found not to be in compliance. The cost of this testing is currently paid by the government agency. By cooperating in this program, the retailers are able to check the residue status of the products they market without duplicating an existing government program. Thus, the objectives of both government and industry to ensure the safety of food products are met cooperatively.

This is a change from what is often referred to as a "command and control" system. It involves a change from a policing role to an auditing role, where the focus is more on compliance with the regulatory requirement through measures instituted in the industry's quality system rather than with direct inspection of each product. It places the responsibility squarely on the producers of the goods to ensure that they comply with the regulatory requirement.

ANTICIPATING THE FUTURE

While attempts to predict the future frequently are demonstrated by subsequent events to be very different from the eventual reality, perhaps we can attempt to analyze some of the trends that I have discussed and use these to develop our model. In summary, the major change is a shift from inspection of individual goods for defaults to a default prevention system based on HACCP principles, with a resulting change in the role of the government inspector from what we might describe as "quality control", through inspection of individual goods, to "quality assurance", through the auditing of the quality control systems used by industry. This requires a change in attitude from both regulators and industry, moving from what some might see as an adversarial system, to a more cooperative approach. In this new model, the regulators will set the standards and approve the systems used by industry to see that the standards are met. The regulatory authority will, in most cases, apply statistical sampling in auditing the effectiveness of industry control systems. To facilitate this approach, there will be an increasing need for suitable rapid test technology to perform the required tests to keep the production system in control, whether that is a test to ensure that a feed no longer contains a medicating ingredient, a test to ensure that residues have depleted in an animal or in a food commodity prior to harvest, or a test applied at the slaughter or packing facility, or at the retail level, to ensure product compliance. Currently, monitoring systems are used to ensure that products remain within a required temperature range in transit between the food processor and the wholesale or retail level (Curlee 1997). In some cases, we may see developments which will provide a sensor or indicator in the finished product at retail level which will assure the consumer that the product has not been thawed and refrozen, not been exposed to an excess temperature or perhaps even that it does not contain levels of certain microbiological or chemical contaminants which could pose a risk to the consumer. Such technologies are now available, or under development in research laboratories. The next challenge is to have them available at a cost that is acceptable to the consumer.

Thus, the future, at least for the next decade, will perhaps bring a continued evolution toward a total quality system approach, where government sets standards, then assists industry in the development of systems to ensure that their products meet those standards. Government will audit for compliance and government and industry will together work to provide consumers with better means to make informed choices about the safety and quality of the foods that they consume. Put simply, food safety is a shared responsibility, with each sector — producer, regulator, consumer — playing an important and inter-related role.

REFERENCES

Association of Official Analytical Chemists. 1991. AOAC announces new test kit rapid verification program. J. Assoc. Off. Anal. Chem. *74*, 143A.

CLAPP, S. 1997. HACCP offers major opportunities for laboratory managers. Inside Laboratory Management, *1* (2), 17–19.

CURLEE, J. 1997. Monitoring on the move. Food Quality, June/July, 32–37.

FAO. 1993. Codex Alimentarius, Volume 3: Residues of Veterinary Drugs in Foods, 2nd ed. Food and Agriculture Organization of the United Nations, Rome.

Food Inspection Directorate. 1990. Annual Report on Chemical & Biological Testing of Agri-Food Commodities During the Fiscal Year 1989-90. Food Inspection Directorate, Agriculture Canada, Ottawa.

Food Inspection Directorate. 1996. Annual Report on Chemical & Biological Testing of Agri-Food Commodities During the Fiscal Year 1995-96; Vol. 1. Meat Products, Egg Products. Food Inspection Directorate, Agriculture & Agri-Food Canada, Ottawa.

KAY, J. 1997. Food retailer surveillance in the U.K. and cooperation with government. Symposium on Issues in Regulatory Monitoring, Abstract 1104. 111th AOAC International Annual Meeting and Exposition, September 7-11, San Diego, CA.

NEIDERT, E., SASCHENBRECKER, P.W., PATTERSON, J.R. and FESSER, A. 1985. Occurrence of sulfa drug residues in Canadian pork liver. Can. Vet. J., *26*, 282–284.

VAN HOUWELING, C.D. 1981. The magnitude of the sulfa residue problem. JAVMA, *178*, 464–466.

CHAPTER 13

STRATEGIES FOR THE CONTROL OF BSE AND SCRAPIE

MARK ROGERS

Department of Zoology
University College Dublin
Belfield, Dublin 4, Ireland

ABSTRACT

Transmissible Spongiform Encephalopathies, or Prion diseases, are fatal neurodegenerative diseases that affect both humans and animals. Examples include Creutzfeldt-Jakob disease (CJD) in humans, Bovine Spongiform Encephalopathy (BSE) in cattle and scrapie in sheep and goats. They are characterized by a long incubation period, ranging from months to years, and a variable length clinical course, both determined by the particular infection and the species involved. Some 170,000 cattle in the UK have been diagnosed with BSE and have been destroyed. In the rest of Europe there have also been cases of BSE, though the numbers involved are much lower. The recent potential link between BSE and a new variant form of CJD has highlighted the importance of controlling both BSE and scrapie in Ireland. Control of the disease in both cattle and sheep is complicated by the long incubation period, the lack of suitable tests and the general lack of detailed information in relation to the biology of the disease. Factors that must be considered in designing an effective control strategy include (1) better understanding of the epidemiology of the disease, (2) developing rapid and reliable tests for the disease, (3) introducing a suitable surveillance system for both BSE and scrapie, (4) minimising the consequences for farmers that have BSE-infected animals, and (5) implementing and monitoring legislation to prohibit the spread of potentially infectious material. Each of these areas is discussed and it is proposed that the introduction of best available technology in both the diagnosis and surveillance of the national herd could form the basis for an effective programme against animal prion diseases.

BACKGROUND

Bovine spongiform encephalopathy (BSE) and scrapie are examples of transmissible spongiform encephalopathies (TSEs) or prion diseases. These diseases share a number of common features including long-incubation periods and progressive neurological degeneration ending in death. The observed pathology includes characteristic spongiform changes in the brain often associated with the deposition of an amyloidogenic protein called PrP^{res} or PrP^{Sc} (DeArmond and Prusiner 1995). Table 1 details the major human and animal prion diseases.

TABLE 1.
MAJOR HUMAN AND ANIMAL PRION DISEASES

'Natural' Host	TSE / Prion Agent
Human	Creutzfeldt-Jakob disease (CJD) Gerstmann-Sträussler-Scheinker (GSS) Fatal Familial Insomnia (FFI) Kuru
Sheep / Goats	Scrapie
Mink	Transmissible Mink Encephalopathy (TME)
Cattle	Bovine Spongiform Encephalopathy (BSE)
Deer / Elk	Chronic Wasting Disease
Cats	Feline Spongiform Encephalopathy (FSE)
Kudu / Nyala / Oryx / Gemsbok / Eland	Spongiform Encephalopathy in captive exotic ungulates

BOVINE SPONGIFORM ENCEPHALOPATHY

The Source of BSE

The original source of the agent responsible for BSE remains unknown, but two hypotheses have been suggested. The first, and perhaps more likely, suggests that cattle were exposed to the scrapie agent (endemic is some sheep flocks) in ruminant-derived protein supplements (Wilesmith *et al.* 1991). Whereas the scrapie agent had previously been inactivated by the rendering process, changes in that process implemented in the 1970s and 1980s led to cattle being exposed to scrapie-contaminated meat and bone meal. Once transmission from sheep to cattle appeared, the 'cattle-adapted scrapie' or BSE was passed between cattle via ruminant-derived protein feed and the BSE epidemic began. The alternative hypothesis suggests that a BSE-like disease has always been present in the cattle population at a low incidence (perhaps 1 in a million), but a thermostable variant of this agent capable of surviving the altered conditions of rendering appeared and spread rapidly through the cattle population via contaminated feed.

The BSE Agent

The nature of the agent causing transmissible spongiform encephalopathies has yet to be defined. A variety of hypotheses have been proposed to describe the agent; none can fully explain all the unusual properties of the agent.

There is broad agreement that a component of the infectious agent is a normal protein (the prion protein) found in the nervous tissue of all mammals (Prusiner and Scott 1997). This protein assumes a typical conformation in animals not incubating BSE; however, animals that are incubating the disease have, in addition to the normal protein, an altered form of the prion protein called PrP^{res}. Many experts in the field suggest that the infectious agent is composed solely of this abnormal protein and there is much evidence to support this view. Others argue that the 'protein only' hypothesis cannot explain some of the properties of the agent, in particular the number of distinct strains of scrapie found both in experimental disease forms in mice and in 'natural' scrapie in sheep. To account for these strains, an agent-specific informational molecule is essential and this would conventionally require a nucleic acid genome of some form.

BSE is a fatal disease of the nervous system in cattle and was initially observed in the UK in 1985 (Wells *et al.* 1987). It has since been diagnosed in cattle in several countries including Ireland where the first case was reported in 1989. To date (March 1998), a total of 284 cases of BSE have been confirmed in the Republic of Ireland and 1758 cases in Northern Ireland (Nov. 1997). This compares with 170,734 cases in Britain (Feb. 1998). The confirmed incidence of BSE in various countries in 1997 is given in Table 2. Belgium is the most recent country to have declared a case of BSE.

TABLE 2.
CONFIRMED INCIDENCE OF BSE IN VARIOUS COUNTRIES IN 1997*

Country	No. of BSE Cases per Million Cattle
United Kingdom	350
Portugal	24
Switzerland	22
Ireland	10
France	0.3

*(Department of Agriculture and Food and OIE)

The disease is caused by a transmissible agent which has been detected in the brain and spinal cord of naturally infected animals and also in the distal ileum, optic nerve, dorsal root ganglia and bone marrow of cattle experimentally challenged with BSE. The infectious agent has not been detected in any other tissues which have been tested in transmission experiments on laboratory rodents.

CONTROL STRATEGIES FOR BSE AND SCRAPIE

There are two main objectives in the development and implementation of a control strategy for animal TSE agents; firstly, to protect human health and, secondly, to eradicate the diseases from the animal population.

Protecting Human Health

Since BSE was recognised in the late 1980s as a TSE disease, the UK and some European countries have carried out surveillance on CJD cases with a view to defining any trends that might have been due to the BSE epidemic. Table 3 shows the figures for human TSE diseases in the UK between 1985 and 1997.

TABLE 3.
INCIDENCE OF TSE DISEASES IN HUMANS IN THE UK, 1985-1997[1]

Year	Referrals	Sporadic	Iatrogenic	Familial	GSS	nvCJD	Total
1985	-	26	1	1	0	-	28
1986	-	26	0	0	0	-	26
1987	-	23	0	0	1	-	24
1988	-	22	1	1	0	-	24
1989	-	28	2	2	0	-	32
1990	53	28	5	0	0	-	33
1991	75	32	1	3	0	-	36
1992	96	44	2	4	1	-	51
1993	78	38	4	2	2	-	46
1994	116	51	1	4	3	-	59
1995	86	34	4	2	3	3	46
1996	134	41	4	2	4	10	61
1997	156	53	6	3	0	10	72

[1] UK Department of Health web site http://www.coi.gov.uk/coi/depts/GDH/GDH.html

While there has been an overall increase in the number of CJD cases observed, this was attributed to an ascertainment bias; however, a new form of CJD with a different clinical presentation and pathology was identified in 1996 (Will *et al.* 1996). This led to the announcement, in March 1996, of a possible link between BSE and the new form of the human Creutzfeldt-Jakob disease (nvCJD) and highlighted the need to develop controls that would protect human health. To date, 23 individuals in the UK and 1 in France have died from nvCJD and the evidence that nvCJD and BSE are caused by the same agent is overwhelming (Bruce *et al.* 1997; Collinge *et al.* 1996; Raymond *et al.* 1997).

To prevent BSE-infected meat or meat products entering the food chain, all animals suspected of infection with BSE or scrapie are excluded and all tissues that are potential sources of infectious agent are removed from all animals. This material, designated the 'specified risk material' is described in Table 4.

TABLE 4.
SPECIFIED RISK MATERIAL (SRM) IN CATTLE AND SHEEP

Animal	Age	Tissue
Bovine	>12 months	Skull, Brain, Spinal cord, Eyes
Goat / Sheep	permanent incisor tooth	Skull, Brain, Spinal cord, Eyes
Sheep	all	Spleen

This procedure has been adopted to ensure that tissues from animals that may be incubating the disease, but which show no clinical signs, are removed and do not enter the human or animal food chain. It is likely that all individuals who have died of nvCJD contracted the disease from the consumption of BSE-contaminated meat and meat products prior to the implementation of the ban on the use of these tissues. The uncertainties in the effectiveness of the UK ban, the length of the incubation period of nvCJD, and the level of exposure of the population to the agent make an assessment of the potential total number of nvCJD cases impossible; however, estimates range from a low of tens of cases, to a high of tens of thousands of cases.

Eradication of Animal TSEs

The main strategy in place to prevent the spread of and to eliminate BSE has been to control the known routes of transmission of the disease. Epidemiological investigations in the UK have identified the main cause of infection in cattle as exposure to contaminated ruminant-derived meat and bone meal used as a protein supplement. The use of ruminant-derived meat and bone meal in feed for ruminants was banned in the UK in 1989 and in Ireland in 1990. The long incubation period of the disease in cattle, on average 4 to 5 years, meant that the effect of these bans would not be observed until 1994 or 1995; however, cattle born after the implementation of these bans in both countries have subsequently been infected indicating that this ban was not completely effective. This was probably due to old stocks of feed containing ruminant-derived meat and bone meal, and poor compliance with implementation of the ban as well as problems of cross-contamination in the feed industry. It was common practice to use the same production line to produce pig and poultry feed (where ruminant-derived meat and bone meal was allowed) on one day and subsequently to produce cattle feed. Since it is impractical to ensure that the production line was free from ruminant proteins, cross-contamination could occur.

Recently, new legislation has been put in place which requires premises that will produce, sell, store or use ruminant-derived meat and bone meal to be licensed. No license is granted for the handling of ruminant meat and bone meal to a premises where products for cattle are also produced, sold, stored or used. This stringent regulation, if properly enforced, should result in the elimination of any potential cross-contamination with BSE-infected material.

The second route of transmission of BSE that has been identified is maternal transmission. There is a small risk that a calf born from a dam that is within 6 months of showing clinical signs of BSE will also contract the disease. The level of transmission by this route is too small to maintain the disease in the population in the absence of other modes of transmission.

Surveillance

In Ireland, BSE and scrapie are notifiable diseases and the main mechanism of surveillance currently is through this legislation. Animals suspected of having BSE or scrapie are notified to the Department of Agriculture and Food and the herd or flock is restricted. In the case of BSE, the suspect animal is slaughtered *in situ* and the brain is sent to the Veterinary Research Laboratory for diagnosis. The carcass is buried on the farm. If BSE is confirmed, the remainder of the herd is sent for slaughter at a designated factory and the carcasses rendered and incinerated. An extensive epidemiological investigation is carried out to determine the history of the BSE case and any progeny or cohort animals identified, traced and slaughtered. The brains of these animals are also examined for signs of BSE. To date, approximately 9,000 cohort animals have been slaughtered and 5 preclinical cases of BSE identified.

A surveillance strategy which relies on the diagnosis of BSE by veterinary practitioners begs the question whether all cases of BSE are being detected. While the answer to this is unclear, the ratio of reported versus confirmed cases of BSE gives some information. Figure 1 shows the number of reported versus confirmed cases over the period 1989 to 1996.

Between 1989 and 1996, approximately half the reported cases of BSE have subsequently been confirmed. The overall low incidence of the disease in Ireland makes any analysis of these numbers difficult, but the high ratio of reported versus confirmed cases suggests that suspect cases are being referred for investigation; however, the observation of an increase in the number of reported cases which parallels the number of confirmed cases may be indicative of some under-reporting in the past.

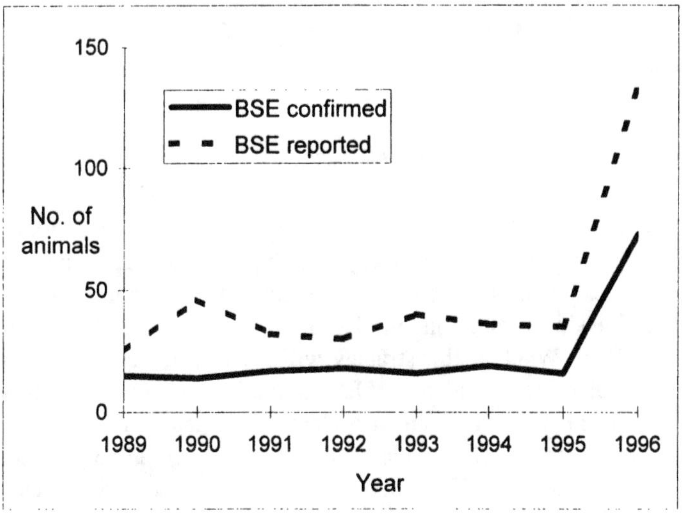

FIG. 1. REPORTED VERSUS CONFIRMED CASES OF BSE IN IRELAND, 1989-1996 (data from the Irish Department of Agriculture and Food, available at http://www.irlgov.ie/)

Diagnosis

One of the major problems in detecting BSE is the method of diagnosis for the disease. Currently diagnosis is made by a postmortem histological examination of the brain for the presence of classic pathology associated with the disease. To date, no test for the diagnosis of BSE or scrapie in the live animal exists though a test for BSE has been developed which can detect disease in the carcass. The lack of tissues from preclinical animals has precluded the validation of this test in the diagnosis of disease in preclinical animals; however, it is reasonable to assume that the test would detect the disease in animals which are preclinical, but show pathology on postmortem examination. As such, the test would be more sensitive than current methods of diagnosis at abattoirs, which are based solely on clinical signs. The importance of detecting animals at this stage of the disease (shortly before clinical signs) has recently been highlighted by the discovery of detectable levels of infectious agent in the dorsal root ganglia of animals experimentally infected with BSE but which were between 2 and 7 months preclinical.

The low incidence of the disease and the policy of slaughtering of the entire herd when a case is confirmed makes the use of such a test problematic as even a test with high specificity may identify some animals as being BSE-positive when they are not. Such identification would result in serious costs associated with compensation to farmers. The implementation of this test on a large-scale basis might require a reevaluation of the whole herd slaughter policy for animals shown positive by the test, but for which no pathology is found on postmortem examination.

CONCLUSION

The incidence of BSE in Ireland is low and the stringent legislation in force to protect the consumer from potentially infected food should provide confidence regarding the safety of Irish beef. New legislation to regulate the supply of ruminant-derived meat and bone meal should, over time, lead to a drop in the incidence of BSE. Whether this strategy will result in the eventual elimination of BSE or whether a low incidence of BSE in the European beef sector will have to be tolerated remains to be seen. It is clear that legislation is effective only if it is strictly enforced. The implementation of a surveillance scheme that examines the cattle and sheep populations for disease independent of the eradication scheme would seem prudent if an objective assessment of the eradication scheme is to be made.

REFERENCES

BRUCE, M.E. *et al.* 1997. Transmissions to mice indicate that 'new variant' CJD is caused by the BSE agent. Nature *389*, 498–501.

COLLINGE, J., SIDLE, K.C., MEADS, J., IRONSIDE, J. and HILL, A.F. 1996. Molecular analysis of prion strain variation and the aetiology of 'new variant' CJD. Nature *383*, 685–690.

DEARMOND, S.J. and PRUSINER, S.B. 1995. Etiology and pathogenesis of prion diseases. Am. J. Pathol. *146*, 785–811.

PRUSINER, S.B. and SCOTT, M.R. 1997. Genetics of prions. Annu. Rev. Genet. *31*, 75–139.

RAYMOND, G.J. *et al.* 1997. Molecular assessment of the potential transmissibilities of BSE and scrapie to humans. Nature *388*, 285–288.

WELLS, G.A.H. *et al.* 1987. A Novel progressive Spongiform Encephalopathy in cattle. Vet Rec *121*, 419–420.

WILESMITH, J.W., RYAN, J.B. and ATKINSON, M.J. 1991. Bovine Spongiform Encephalopathy: Epidemiological studies on the origin. Vet. Rec. *128*, 199–203.

WILL, R.G. 1996. A new variant of Creutzfeldt-Jakob disease in the UK. Lancet *347*, 921–925.

CHAPTER 14

INACTIVATION OF THE BSE AGENT

D. M. TAYLOR

Neuropathogenesis Unit
Institute for Animal Health
West Mains Road
Edinburgh EH9 3JF
UK

ABSTRACT

Bovine spongiform encephalopathy (BSE) belongs to a distinct group of transmissible degenerative encephalopathies (TDE) that includes scrapie in sheep and Creutzfeldt-Jakob disease (CJD) of humans. These fatal neurological diseases are caused by unconventional but uncharacterised transmissible agents that have a number of unusual properties; this includes a high degree of resistance to inactivation. The only disinfectant that appears to be completely effective against high titres of TDE infectivity is sodium hypochlorite. Exposure to 1 to 2 M sodium hydroxide has a substantial but incomplete effect, as does autoclaving at temperatures between 132 and 138C for up to an hour; however, a combination of 2 M sodium hydroxide and autoclaving, even at the more modest temperature of 121C for 30 min, appears to be completely effective. With lower titres of infectivity, less rigorous regimes may be effective. For example, although most of the rendering procedures used to manufacture meat and bone meal (MBM) throughout the European Union (EU) have been found to be incapable of inactivating BSE and scrapie agents, one method which appeared to be effective with moderate titres of BSE and scrapie agent, involved exposure to steam at 133C for 20 min. This procedure is now the only one approved within the EU for the manufacture of MBM for feeding animals, excluding ruminants; however, the UK has introduced a ban on feeding MBM to any farmed species because of the occurrence of a new variant form of CJD in the UK which appears to have been caused by the BSE agent.

Although the clinical signs of scrapie in sheep are entirely attributable to neurological dysfunction, tissues such as spleen and lymph nodes are known to become infected before those of the central nervous system. In contrast, the only tissues which have been found to become infected in cattle with natural BSE are brain, spinal cord and retina. These are no longer used in animal or human foodstuff. Because scrapie agent has no known association with human disease there has been no restriction in the past on using any sheep tissues, including brain, as human food; however, it is known from experimental studies that the BSE agent can infect sheep by the oral route to cause a disease that is clinically and neurohistopathologically indistinguishable from scrapie. It is also known that the spleen becomes infected in such sheep. Sheep in the UK could theoretically have become infected with the BSE agent through the feeding of infected MBM before the feed-ban in 1988. There are now measures in place that prevent the head, spinal cord, and spleen of sheep being incorporated into foodstuff.

INTRODUCTION

The transmissible degenerative encephalopathies (TDE) form a group of unusual neurological diseases which includes scrapie in sheep, bovine spongiform encephalopathy (BSE), and Creutzfeldt-Jakob disease (CJD) of humans. The incidence of BSE in the UK is now declining rapidly, but concern regarding this disease has been heightened by its putative link with a new variant form of CJD which was first reported in 1996 (Will *et al.* 1996). The probability that this new form of CJD is caused by the BSE agent was made even more likely by the data of Bruce *et al.* (1997). These showed that the phenotypic characteristics of this agent were exactly the same as those of the BSE agent which, in turn, is quite unlike any other TDE agent that has yet been characterised. Although the unconventional transmissible agents which cause TDE have not yet been characterised, it has been recognised for some time that they have a relatively high degree of resistance to decontamination procedures that are effective with conventional microorganisms e.g. exposure to potassium permanganate, phenolic disinfectants (Kimberlin *et al.* 1983), and peracetic acid (Taylor 1991). As a consequence of their resistance to inactivation, these agents have been responsible for the accidental transmission of TDE. CJD has been transmitted accidentally through the use of inadequately decontaminated neurosurgical equipment (Bernoulli *et al.* 1977; Foncin *et al.* 1980). Scrapie has been transmitted accidentally through the failure to inactivate the agent in a vaccine (Greig 1950). BSE was considered to have been transmitted accidentally through survival of infectivity after the cooking procedures used to manufacture meat and bone for inclusion in animal feeds (Wilesmith *et al.* 1988), and the general failure of these processes to completely inactivate BSE and scrapie agents has been demonstrated (Taylor *et al.* 1995; 1997b). Despite these problems, it was considered by the late 1980s that a few reliable decontamination procedures for TDE agents had been established. In the UK, the recommended methods were porous-load (PL) autoclaving at 134-138C for 18 min (DHSS 1984), or exposure to sodium hypochlorite solution containing 20,000 ppm available chlorine for an hour (Kimberlin *et al.* 1983). The preference in the USA was to use gravity-displacement (GD) autoclaving at

132C for an hour, or exposure to 1M sodium hydroxide for an hour (Rosenberg *et al.* 1986). These various recommended procedures were adopted worldwide. In the 1990s, further decontamination studies on BSE and scrapie agents were initiated, and these will be discussed. The source of the BSE agent was infected cow-brain; the scrapie agents were hamster- or mouse-passaged strains. The assays for residual infectivity were carried out by intracerebral injection of the samples into hamsters or mice. Where the amount of residual infectivity was to be measured, serial dilutions were injected. Intracerebral injection is the most sensitive route for bioassay of these agents; however, when transmission is across a species barrier, such as cow to mouse in the case of BSE, there is a reduction in the efficiency of transmission. It has been shown that assaying BSE infectivity by intracerebral injection of mice is around 1,000-fold less sensitive than intracerebral assay in cattle (Ministry of Agriculture Fisheries and Food, personal communication).

Chemical Methods

There was little reduction in BSE infectivity after a two-year exposure to formol saline (Fraser *et al.* 1992). This was not surprising, given that TDE agents are known generally to resist inactivation by formalin and other aldehydes (Taylor 1992). BSE infectivity was inactivated by exposure for 30 min to solutions of sodium hypochlorite containing up to 16,500 ppm available chlorine (Taylor *et al.* 1994). In contrast, solutions of sodium dichloroisocyanurate with equivalent concentrations of available chlorine were not effective, even after 2-h treatments due to the reluctance of this chemical to yield its available chlorine content (Taylor *et al.* 1994). Studies with BSE-infected bovine brain and scrapie-infected rodent brain showed that treatment with 1 or 2 M sodium hydroxide for up to 2 h did not completely inactivate these agents, and permitted the survival of up to four logs of infectivity (Taylor *et al.* 1994). This finding appears to contradict earlier data which showed that a 1-h treatment with 1 M sodium hydroxide was effective (Brown *et al.* 1986). In the earlier study the sensitivity of the bioassay was reduced considerably by the need to dilute the samples before injection; however, in the more recent study, it was not found necessary to dilute the samples. There have also been other reports that sodium hydroxide is not a completely reliable disinfectant for TDE agents (Ernst and Race 1993).

Heat Treatment

Scrapie agent was not inactivated by microwave irradiation (Taylor and Diprose 1996) or dry heat at temperatures of up to 180C for an hour (Taylor *et al.* 1996b); there was even some survival of infectivity after exposure at 160C for 24 h but a 1-h exposure at 200C was effective. This appears not to support other data showing some survival of infectivity after exposure to 360C for an hour (Brown *et al.* 1990); however, lyophilized tissue was used in the latter study; prior drying is known to enhance the thermostability of conventional microorganisms and TDE agents (Asher *et al.* 1986; 1987).

Undiluted macerates (350 mg) and saline homogenates of BSE-infected bovine brain were exposed to GD autoclaving at 132C. Survival of infectivity in both types of sample after a 30-min exposure was not surprising, given that CJD and scrapie agents had been shown previously to survive after a thirty, but not sixty, minute exposure (Brown *et al.* 1986). After a 60-min exposure the BSE-infected macerate, but not the homogenate, was still infectious; however, there is the unanswered question as to whether or not 350-mg samples of infected, undiluted brain represent an excessive challenge for GD autoclaves. Nevertheless, others have reported some survival of scrapie infectivity after infected brain homogenates were exposed to GD autoclaving at 132C for an hour (Pocchiari 1993; Ernst and Race 1993). Samples (340 mg) of macerated BSE-infected bovine brain and scrapie-infected rodent brain were subjected to PL autoclaving at 134-138C for periods of up to an hour; none of the cycles produced complete inactivation (Taylor *et al.* 1994). These results appear to clash with earlier data showing inactivation by PL autoclaving at 136C for 4 min (Kimberlin *et al.* 1983); however, the sample sizes in the earlier study were smaller (50 mg). The degree of smearing and drying onto the glass containers that occurred with the larger (340 mg) samples was considered to be the main explanation for the survival of infectivity in these samples, as discussed above. It may be argued that partial drying of infectivity onto glass or metal surfaces should be a prerequisite when trying to define effective standards for inactivating TDE agents by heat. Thermostability of TDE agents is also enhanced by prior exposure to formalin (Taylor and McConnell 1988) or ethanol (Taylor 1996b). In contrast, even GD autoclaving at 121C for 30 min appears to be effective if carried out in the presence of, or preceded by treatment with, sodium hydroxide (Taylor *et al.* 1997a).

The kinetics of thermal inactivation of TDE agents is interesting and perplexing. When incomplete inactivation occurs, the inactivation curve tends to show a steep initial decline, and then flatten and persist with time (Rohwer 1983). This indicates that a subfraction of the infectivity is more thermostable, and this appears to represent a fairly constant amount irrespective of the starting titre (Taylor 1996a). Such a phenomenon might be caused by protective aggregation, but this is speculative and unproven.

Modification of the Dose-Response Curve

Under well-defined experimental conditions specific strains of scrapie agent in rodents display highly reproducible inverse relationships between the dose of infectivity administered and the subsequent incubation period before terminal illness occurs. For any given model the amount of infectivity present in an inoculum can be calculated by comparing the incubation period of the recipients with an 'incubation period assay' graph, without the need for titration. Unfortunately this procedure cannot be applied to infectivity exposed to chemical or physical treatments because these can radically extend the dose-response curves for treated, compared with untreated, agent (Taylor *et al.* 1995; Taylor and Fernie 1996; Taylor *et al.* 1996b). This means that a meaningful assessment of the amount of infectivity remaining after exposure to partially inactivating procedures can only be obtained by full titration, and observing the assay animals for extended periods.

Rendering

Epidemiological studies demonstrated an association between BSE and the practice of feeding cattle with meat and bone meal (MBM) manufactured from animal waste (Wilesmith *et al.* 1988). It appeared that the causal agent could survive the heating processes used during manufacture. Experimental, pilot-scale facsimiles of the various production methods for MBM were used to process raw materials spiked with BSE or scrapie agents, and then determine whether infectivity could be detected in the end-products. BSE infectivity was detectable in MBM produced by two types of procedure (Taylor *et al.* 1995). One was a process in which cooking took place at atmospheric pressure over a period of 50 min with the end-temperature reaching either 112 or 122C. The other was conducted under vacuum with added preheated fat, in the form of tallow; exposure times were either 10 or 40 min, and the final temperatures were 120 and 121C, respectively. As a result of these positive findings the minimum conditions for rendering ruminant-derived material within the EU were revised (Commission Decision 1994). The more recent studies on the same rendering processes, using scrapie-spiked raw materials, have shown that MBM produced by all processes (except those involving exposure to pressurized steam) was infected (Taylor *et al.* 1996a; 1997b). Consequently, the only procedure which is now permitted for processing of mammalian raw material into MBM for incorporation into animal diets in the EU involves processing either the raw materials or MBM in steam at a pressure of three bars and a temperature of 133C for at least 20 min (Commission Decision 1996). Although this process inactivated spiked raw materials containing $10^{1.7}$ mouse ID_{50}/g of BSE agent or $10^{3.1}$ ID_{50}/g of scrapie agent, the levels of infectivity that the process may have to cope with in practice may be higher. This is because, although it was necessary to thoroughly mix the BSE and scrapie-infected brains with the raw materials in the rendering experiments, infected brain-tissue will not become distributed throughout the raw materials in this fashion during everyday rendering. This is supported by the frequent occurrence of only one or two cases of BSE in herds of cattle, which indicates that BSE infectivity occurs as pockets in MBM, rather than being evenly distributed throughout infected batches. The titre of infectivity in individual brains from BSE-infected cattle can be greater than 10^5 ID_{50}/g (Fraser *et al.* 1992) which is almost 3 logs higher than the level tested in the rendering experiments. Similarly, the level of infectivity in the brains of sheep with scrapie can reach 10^6 ID_{50}/g overall, and be as high as 10^8 $ID_{50}50/g$ in specific areas of the brain (Hadlow *et al.* 1979). These levels are 3-5 logs higher than those achieved in the scrapie-spiked rendering experiments. The idea that the rendering process involving steam at 133C for 20 min may not be entirely reliable under worst-case conditions is supported by experimental data which show survival of BSE infectivity in 340 mg samples of infected cattle-brain (with an infectivity titre of $10^{3\text{-}5}$ ID_{50}/g) after autoclaving at 132C for an hour (referred to in the previous section); however, it has to be acknowledged that the conditions of exposure were such that smearing and drying of the infected brain-tissue onto surfaces could have occurred before autoclaving, and this would not occur during rendering. Other data obtained from the use of saline homogenates of scrapie-infected hamster brain avoid such complications, and demonstrate survival of some infectivity following autoclaving at 132 or 134C for an hour; these data are referred to in the previous section. The overall conclusion is that if BSE or scrapie-infected brain and (possibly) sheep spleens are rendered by the 133C steam process, there may be infectivity in the resulting MBM (Taylor 1997). Recent studies, using a higher titre of BSE infectivity than before, have shown that infectivity can survive the 133C process (Schreuder *et al.* 1988). In view of the concern that the cases of new variant CJD in Britain may be causally linked with BSE through dietary exposure, the use of MBM in the diet of any farmed animal species has been prohibited in the UK.

Although it seems likely that BSE was caused initially by scrapie agent, no strain of scrapie agent with the same phenotypic characteristics as BSE agent has ever been recovered from sheep. This does not rule out the possibility that BSE was caused originally by scrapie agent because there has been only a limited number of primary transmissions of scrapie from sheep to mice. It is possible that a single, previously-uncharacterised, strain of scrapie agent has the capacity to preferentially cross the bovine species-barrier. It is also possible that the strain of scrapie that caused BSE happened to be selected out by the rendering process because it is more thermostable than other strains. Alternatively, the BSE agent may have had a bovine origin. In the scrapie-spiked rendering studies, infected MBM was produced by two processes that achieved the relatively high temperature of 138C, and transmission studies are underway with these two MBM samples to determine whether the pattern of incubation periods and brain-lesion profiles produced in five strains of mice is similar to that of the

BSE agent, as described by Bruce and others (1994). Given that the scrapie-infected brain-pool used as the spike came from 2,867 sheep distributed throughout England, Scotland and Wales, it seems likely that if BSE was caused originally by scrapie agent, the strain responsible would be present in this brain-pool.

It has been postulated that the abandonment of solvent extraction in the UK, as an adjunct to rendering, by the early 1980s may have been a factor which permitted BSE to emerge in the mid 1980s (Wilesmith *et al.* 1988). Traditionally, greaves (the solid product remaining after standard rendering procedures) had commonly been subjected to solvent extraction to enhance the yield of tallow, and produce a low-fat MBM which had attracted premium prices. The notion has been that the exposure to hot solvents and/or the heat treatments used to drive off residual solvent may have been sufficient to keep infectivity levels in MBM below the effective oral dose for cattle. In the scrapie-spiked rendering studies, infected greaves were subjected to solvent extraction with hot heptane. After draining, the greaves were exposed to steam to drive off residual solvent. Although the level of infectivity in the rendered tissue, before solvent extraction, was low, infectivity was still recoverable after treatment with heptane, or heptane followed by steam-treatment (Taylor *et al.* 1997b). Quantitative laboratory studies on four solvent extraction systems have shown only a small degree in the reduction of BSE or scrapie infectivity (Taylor *et al.* 1998).

There is no rational scientific reason why MBM should not be fed to any species within which it is nutritionally useful, provided that the manufacturing process can consistently inactivate not only conventional pathogenic agents such as *Salmonella* species but also TDE agents that might be present in the raw materials; however, the emotional, ethical and political implications of the BSE saga are unlikely to allow this to happen in the near future. Nevertheless, new rendering processes which offer the potential of an even greater degree of reassurance regarding the safety of the MBM end-product are being assessed. If these processes live up to expectations, there may be a case for allowing MBM to be fed once again to ruminants and (in the UK) other farmed species.

REFERENCES

ASHER, D.C., POMEROY, K.L, MURPHY, L., ROHWER, R.G., GIBBS, C.J. and GAJDUSEK, D.C. 1986. Practical inactivation of scrapie agent on surfaces. Abstracts of the IXth International Congress of Infectious and Parasitic Diseases, Munich 1986.

ASHER, D.M., POMEROY, K.L., MURPHY, L., GIBBS, C.J. and GAJDUSEK, D.C. 1987. Attempts to disinfect surfaces contaminated with etiological agents of the spongiform encephalopathies. Abstracts of the VIIth International Congress of Virology, August 9-14, p. 147, Edmonton.

BERNOULLI, C. *et al.* 1977. Danger of accidental person-to-person transmission of Creutzfeld-Jakob disease by surgery. Lancet *i*, 478–479.

BROWN, P., LIBERSKI, P.P., WOLFF, A. and GAJDUSEK, D.C. 1990. Resistance of scrapie agent to steam autoclaving after formaldehyde fixation and limited survival after ashing at 360C: practical and theoretical implications. J. Infect. Dis. *161*, 467–472.

BROWN, P., ROHWER, R.G. and GAJDUSEK, D.C. 1986. Newer data on the inactivation of scrapie virus or Creutzfeldt-Jakob disease virus in brain tissue. J. Infect. Dis. *153*, 1145–1148.

BRUCE, M.E., CHREE, A., McCONNELL, I., FOSTER, J., PEARSON, G. and FRASER, H. 1994. Transmission of bovine spongiform encephalopathy and scrapie to mice; strain variation and the species barrier. Philosophical Trans. Royal Soc. B *343*, 405–411.

BRUCE, M.E. *et al.* 1997. Transmissions to mice indicate that 'new variant' CJD is caused by the BSE agent. Lancet *389*, 498–501.

Commission Decision 1994. On the approval of alternative heat treatment systems for processing animal waste of ruminant origin with a view to the inactivation of spongiform encephalopathy agents. Commission Decision 941382/EC. Official J. Eur. Comm. *L172*, 25–27.

Commission Decision 1996. On the approval of alternative heat treatment systems for processing animal waste with a view to the inactivation of spongiform encephalopathy agents. Commission Decision 96/449/EC. Official J. Eur. Comm. *L184*, 43–46.

DHSS 1984. Management of patients with spongiform encephalopathy (Creutzfeldt-Jakob disease {CJD}). DHSS Circular DA (84) 16.

ERNST, D.R. and RACE, R.E. 1993. Comparative analysis of scrapie agent inactivation. J. Virol. Meth. *41*, 193–202.

FONCIN, J.F., GACHES, J., CATHALA, F., EL SHERIF, E. and LE BEAU 1980. Transmission iatrogene interhumaine possible de maladie de Creutzfeldt-Jakob avec alteinte des grains du cervulet. Revue Neurologique *136*, 280.

FRASER, H., BRUCE, M.E., CHREE, A., MCCONNELL, I. and WELLS, G.A.H. 1992. Transmission of bovine spongiform encephalopathy and scrapie to mice. J. Gen. Virol. *173*, 1891–1897.

GREIG, J.R. 1950. Scrapie in sheep. J. Comp. Pathology *60*, 263-266.

HADLOW, W.J., RACE, R.E., KENNEDY, R.C. and EKLUND, C.M. 1979. Natural infection of sheep with scrapie virus. In *Transmissible Slow Diseases of the Nervous System*. Vol. 2. (S.B. Prusiner and W.J. Hadlow, eds.) pp. 3–12, Academic Press, London.

KIMBERLIN, R.H. *et al.* 1983. Disinfection studies with two strains of mouse-passaged scrapie agent. J. Neurol. Sci. *59*, 355–369.

POCCHIARI, M. Unpublished data cited by HORAUD, F. 1993. Safety of medicinal products: summary. Developments in Biological Standardisation *80*, 207–208.

ROHWER, R.G. 1983. Scrapie inactivation kinetics - an explanation for scrapie's apparent resistance to inactivation - a re-evaluation of estimates of its small size. In *Virus non Conventionnels et Affections du Systeme Nerveux Central* (L.A. Court and F. Cathala, eds.) pp. 84– 113, Masson, Paris.

ROSENBERG, R.N. *et al.* 1986. Precautions in handling tissues, fluids, and other contaminated materials from patients with documented or suspected Creutzfeldt-Jakob disease. Annals Neurol. *19*, 75–77.

SCHREUDER, B.E.C. *et al.* 1998. Studies on the efficacy of hyperbaric rendering procedures in inactivating bovine spongiform encephalopathy (BSE) and scrapie agents. Vet. Record *142*, 474-480.

TAYLOR, D.M. 1991. Resistance of the ME7 scrapie agent to peracetic acid. Vet. Microbiol. *27*, 19–24.

TAYLOR, D.M. 1992. Inactivation of unconventional agents of the transmissible degenerative encephalopathies. In *Principles and Practice of Disinfection Preservation and Sterilization* (A.D. Russel, W.B. Hugo and G.A.J. Ayliffe, eds.) pp. 171–179, Blackwell Scientific Publications, Oxford.

TAYLOR, D.M. 1996a. Creutzfeldt-Jakob disease. Lancet *347*, 1333.

TAYLOR, D.M. 1996b. Transmissible subacute spongiform encephalopathies: Practical aspects of agent inactivation. In *Transmissible Subacute Spongiform Encephalopathies: Prion Diseases* (L. Court and E. Dodet, eds.) pp. 479–482, Elsevier, Paris.

TAYLOR, D.M. 1997. Research on the safety of meat and bone meal with regard to bovine spongiform encephalopathy and scrapie agents. July 1–2, Trans. Intl. Conf. on Meat and Bone Meal, pp. 37–40; 42–44; 63. Brussels.

TAYLOR, D.M. and DIPROSE, M.F. 1996. The response of the 22A strain of scrapie agent to microwave irradiation compared with boiling. Neuropathol. Appl. Neurobiol. *22*, 256–258.

TAYLOR, D.M. and FERNIE, K. 1996. Exposure to autoclaving or sodium hydroxide extends the dose-response curve of the 263K strain of scrapie agent in hamsters. J. Gen. Virol. *77*, 811–813.

TAYLOR, D.M., FERNIE, K. and McCONNELL, I. 1997a. Inactivation of the 22A strain of scrapie agent by autoclaving in sodium hydroxide. Vet. Microbiol. *58*, 87–91.

TAYLOR, D.M., FERNIE, K., McCONNELL, FERGUSON, C.E. and STEELE, P. 1998. Solvent extraction as an adjunct to rendering; the effect on BSE and scrapie agents of hot solvents, followed by dry heat and steam. Vet. Record *143*, 6–9.

TAYLOR, D.M. 1994. Decontamination studies with the agents of bovine spongiform encephalopathy and scrapie. Arch. Virol. *139*, 313–326.

TAYLOR, D.M. and McCONNELL, I. 1988. Autoclaving does not decontaminate formol fixed scrapie tissues. Lancet *i*, 1463–1464.

TAYLOR, D.M., McCONNELL, I. and FERNIE, K. 1996b. The effect of dry heat on the ME7 strain of scrapie agent. J. Gen. Virol. *77*, 3161- 3164.

TAYLOR, D.M., WOODGATE, S.L. and ATKINSON, M.J. 1995. Inactivation of the bovine spongiform encephalopathy agent by rendering procedures. Vet. Record *137*, 605–610.

TAYLOR, D.M., WOODGATE, S.L. and FLEETWOOD, A.J. 1996a. Scrapie agent survives rendering procedures. p. 33, Abstracts of the Jubilee Meeting of the Assoc. Veterinary Teachers and Res. Workers, Scarborough.

TAYLOR, D.M., WOODGATE, S.W., FLEETWOOD, A.J. and CAWTHORNE, R.J.G. 1997b. The effect of rendering procedures on scrapie agent. Vet. Record *141*, 643–649.

WILESMITH, J.W., WELLS, G.A.J., CRANWELL, M.P. and RYAN, J.B.M. 1988. Bovine spongiform encephalopathy: epidemiological studies. Vet. Record *123*, 638–644.

WILL, R.G. *et al.* 1996. A new variant form of Creutzfeldt-Jakob disease in the UK. Lancet *347*, 921–925.

CHAPTER 15

HACCP — PRESENT STATUS IN FOOD SAFETY CONTROL

TOM DOYLE

Teagasc, The National Food Centre
Dunsinea, Castleknock, Dublin 15, Ireland

ABSTRACT

The paper reviews the present status of HACCP in the Irish food industry and discusses the level of application of such systems, the perceived benefits or disadvantages and the obstacles to their implementation. The presentation also discusses how HACCP can be integrated with other quality improvement initiatives such as Total Quality Management (TQM), World Class Manufacturing (WCM) and ISO 9000. An assessment is made of the training and advisory services that should be developed to meet the needs of food businesses.

INTRODUCTION

This paper is based on a survey carried out by The National Food Centre in September of 1997 on the level of implementation of HACCP in the Irish food industry. The basic purpose of the survey was to assess the training and advisory needs of food businesses. The National Food Centre has provided food safety and consultancy services to industry for the last ten years but the industry has developed to a point now where there is a need to re-assess what services are required. Six hundred companies were surveyed. The methodology was by confidential questionnaire and one of the initial positive indicators was that there were over two hundred (210) responses to the questionnaire, representing a return rate of approximately 35%. The paper also examines how HACCP is being applied and how it can be used as part of other quality management initiatives in the food industry.

MAIN FINDINGS

In response to the question *"Does your company have a HACCP based food safety control system"* 71% of respondents said yes, 14% indicated that they did not have a system and 15% said they were in the process of developing a system

(Fig. 1). This is in marked contrast to a similar survey that was carried out in 1995 (Connolly 1995). At that time, it was found that only about one-third of food processing companies had HACCP systems in place. A supplementary question was asked relating to when the companies had developed their system, to which 37% indicated within the last year and 37% within the last one to two years. To some extent this response supports the findings of the earlier study.

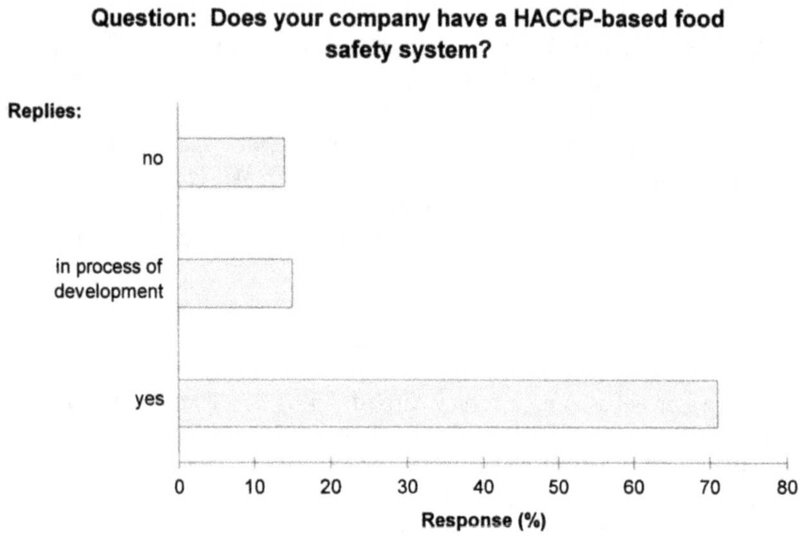

FIG. 1. RESPONSES FROM IRISH FOOD COMPANIES ON THE IMPLEMENTATION OF HACCP

A minimum of five criteria were selected to define a HACCP-based food safety system:

1. Documentation of hygiene procedures.
2. Records of hazard analysis.
3. A HACCP plan.
4. Records of all critical control points (CCPs).
5. Specifications of product, ingredients, raw materials, packaging, etc. available.

Documentation of hygiene procedures was a prerequisite for a HACCP based food safety system. Records of hazard analysis were deliberately included to ascertain if companies actually went through the process of carrying out the hazard analysis themselves, rather than have an "off the shelf" HACCP system, either put in by a consultant or taken from a generic HACCP plan. A HACCP plan, itself, was considered a central requirement and the records of all CCPs were used to establish that there were records that the plan was being followed. Eighty percent of companies were carrying out the hazard analysis themselves.

IMPLEMENTATION BY COMPANY SIZE

The relationship between company size and implementation of HACCP was also studied (Fig. 2). The bigger the company, the more likely it is to have a HACCP system in place. Possible reasons are (a) that large companies are likely to have brands to protect and (b) they have the technical resources to develop HACCP systems. However, even in companies of 1-10 employees there is a positive trend towards developing HACCP systems. It has been the experience of The National Food Centre, in the last year, that small businesses are quite willing to take on the requirements of HACCP if they receive proper guidance. The issue of the kind of training that is required at that level is discussed later in the paper. The author does not subscribe to the theory that there is a threshold in food safety control in terms of company size. If there is legislation for food safety control it should apply across the board. The data in Fig. 2 shows that smaller companies are accepting this principle.

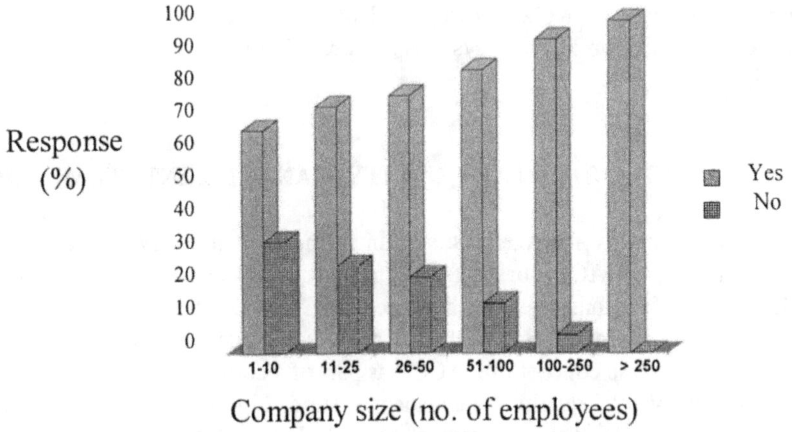

FIG. 2. RELATIONSHIP BETWEEN COMPANY SIZE AND THE IMPLEMENTATION OF A HACCP SYSTEM

Reasons for Implementation

The survey asked companies why they implemented HACCP systems. The most important information was that only 30% of companies cited legal obligations as their prime reason for putting in a HACCP system. Customer demand was listed by 38%, and 32% saw a HACCP system as an internal need for better control. In other words, the companies themselves recognised that HACCP was a useful business process management tool and adopted it as such. The response to supplementary questions about its benefits confirmed this finding. The main conclusion is that the mandatory aspect of HACCP is not the principal motivator. If a food business, or any other organisation, sees a benefit for itself in keeping existing customers or getting new customers or in achieving better internal control within the company it is more likely to develop the system to its full potential.

Reasons for Lack of Implementation

The top three reasons given for not implementing a HACCP system were a lack of knowledge of HACCP, pressure of work and prohibitive financial costs. Personnel in small food businesses can identify with the problems of work pressure and costs, particularly where they do not have the necessary technical resources in terms of quality control personnel that can be committed to developing the systems. Developing hygiene and HACCP systems costs time and money. However, there are programmes, such as the EU Leader programme, which can give assistance.

The National Food Centre has used this programme to assist small food producers in West Cork to develop HACCP systems. The industry development authority, Forbairt, have also recognised the need for state support for small businesses to develop HACCP systems and provide financial assistance for such activities.

HACCP AND TOTAL QUALITY MANAGEMENT (TQM)

A valid quality management system in the food industry is not possible without having a HACCP-based food safety management system. The order of priority for a food business are: hygiene, HACCP, ISO 9000 and then TQM, and this is the successful approach that many companies have taken (Fig. 3).

Turning to the concept of HACCP as part of a company's business process management or total quality management system, Fig. 4 shows the continuous improvement cycle that is common to both HACCP and TQM strategies. Readers familiar with quality assurance will recognise this cycle which is one of the central themes of total quality management.

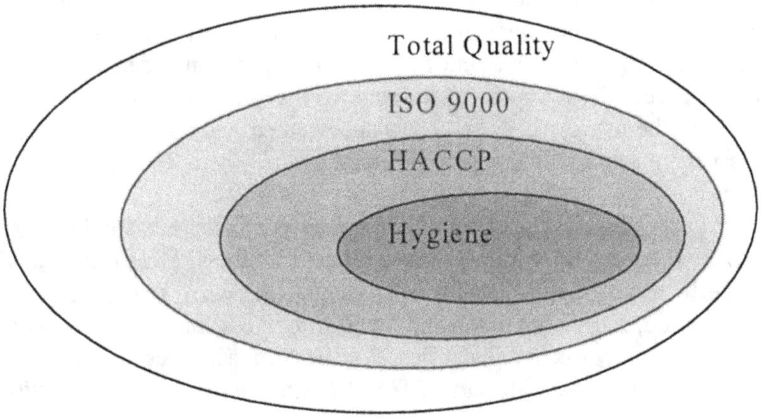

FIG. 3. HACCP AS PART OF A TOTAL QUALITY MANAGEMENT SYSTEM

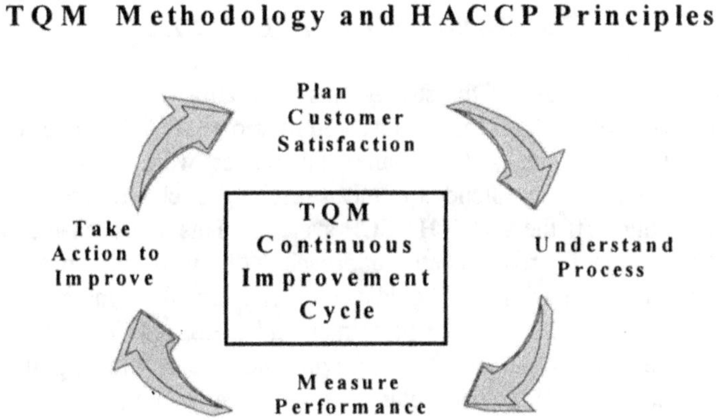

FIG. 4. THE CONTINUOUS IMPROVEMENT CYCLE COMMON TO BOTH HACCP AND TQM STRATEGIES

Essentially, it begins with the customer. In terms of HACCP principles, planning for customer satisfaction means that the food manufacturer must know how the customer uses, and potentially abuses, the product. The food manufacturer must be aware of consumer attitudes to food safety and take them into account when developing products or marketing existing products. The issues of BSE and of growth promoters are examples of real versus perceived risks. The question is not whether these issues give rise to food that is or is not safe but what the consumers want in their meat or other food products.

The continuous improvement cycle, then, requires an understanding of the business process. In terms of understanding the process, HACCP principles require that the process is defined and documented and analysed for hazards. This is very much part of, and complementary to, the approach taken in the application of the principles of total quality management.

Measurement criteria have to be established and there has to be a system of corrective action and improvement within the business. Measuring manufacturing performance for food safety requires deciding what the critical points in the process are, setting the limits and monitoring these limits. Taking action to improve, taking corrective measures, verification activities and monitoring customer complaints are all part of HACCP. In summary, the application of HACCP principles is essentially a first circuit of the TQM cycle. It is intended to use this model to develop TQM programmes for small businesses starting with hygiene and food safety.

The skills that companies learn in developing and documenting HACCP systems should be transferable to other activities in their businesses.

TRAINING AND ADVISORY NEEDS

The main purpose of the survey was to establish the future training and advisory needs of the Irish food industry in relation to HACCP and food safety. The training programmes for smaller businesses were considered to be a priority. Training is not intended to mean teaching in classrooms with manuals and presenting "off-the-shelf" HACCP systems. This approach has been tried and has proved ineffective. A better approach is to give training programmes on an incremental basis with direct guidance on-site. Small businesses do not have quality specialists who can take principles and ideas and develop them into a system. The consultant has to work with the client, drawing up cleaning schedules and hazard control plans. A distance approach will not work. Improved access to hazard data is important. In response to the question, *"Did you have enough scientific data when you were developing your HACCP system?"*, 35% of companies said that they did not. That is a challenge for the regulatory authorities. It is a challenge for organisations like The National Food Centre and it needs to be answered in a way that makes such information easily accessible. There is a need to develop information systems that will allow companies to use modern information technology. This should not be a difficulty with more widespread access to the Internet.

An important dimension of HACCP implementation is the concept of supplier-customer networks. Many of the bigger companies in food processing, catering and retailing have developed an expertise in HACCP systems. This allows them to work with groups of suppliers towards developing HACCP systems. Another contribution to this proceedings (Daly 1998) deals with the approach of working through the food chain to develop food safety management systems at farm level. There is much potential here for co-operation. Some of the big catering organisations in Ireland are already developing supplier-customer networks.

Consultancy and training is also required in the area of internal verification, including audit skills for companies who want to audit their own systems and process validation skills in terms of heat process evaluation, microbiological and challenge testing. There is much demand from regulatory authorities for proof that a process is safe and organisations like The National Food Centre have a role to play. Statistical methods, using the data obtained from a hazard analysis system, applied to development of sampling plans and control charts, provide useful information. Much of the testing carried out in food processing operations could be more efficiently used if statistical methods were applied.

HACCP VERIFICATION

The issue of verification of HACCP systems has yet to be resolved within Ireland. There are developments in verification systems in Europe but a clear picture has not yet emerged. The survey asked companies whether they have external verification; 65% of companies have their system audited by a third party, most frequently by a regulatory authority (43%) and, predictably enough, by retail groups. Companies who had developed HACCP systems indicated that they wanted their systems verified by a third party. They wanted that verification to be knowledgeable and consistent and to be applied across the board to all companies within their sector. Some disquiet has been expressed by companies who had spent time, energy and money developing HACCP systems while competitors who had not developed systems are not subject to regulatory control. There is a need for some formal recognition of companies that have developed acceptable HACCP systems. To some extent this need is addressed under the terms of quality management systems, ISO 9000, and local schemes, such as the Q mark and the Bord Bia Quality Assurance Scheme, in that HACCP is an integral part of these systems. The issue is whether there should be a certification system for HACCP, as such, or a food safety certification system, and what agency would be responsible for such certification. Should it be the regulatory authority, or an organisation like the National Standards Authority of Ireland (NSAI), or private quality associations? Should this certification be carried out purely by inspection, or should it involve product testing and assessment of how customers find the company in terms of product safety? What should the scope of third party verification be? Should other systems within the company be covered, such as the hygiene system, the HACCP system and management review? There is a need for more information about procedures used in other countries for HACCP certification. Food safety certification should be operated on a sectoral basis with a strong scientific input from persons with experience who know the hazards involved in those sectors.

CONCLUSIONS

In summary, the positive finding of the survey is that the food processing industry is using HACCP, and, more importantly, is using it for the right reasons. HACCP is recognised as a means of better process management and of making a business more competitive in meeting customer requirements. HACCP should not be seen as an extra burden but can be the foundation for any Total Quality Management system. In the early days of HACCP, companies who were registered to ISO 9000 asked if this meant they had to 'go round the same block again' and develop another set of documentation. This is not the case. Finally, the survey has given The National Food Centre very useful information on areas for future development in terms of training and consultancy services in food safety.

However, while these data indicate that companies in the food sector will adopt HACCP and will do it successfully, there is no room for complacency. The industry has learned from the experience of ISO 9000 that just developing the system is not enough. It has to be actively used, the principle of continuous improvement has to be applied and the system has to be based on current scientific knowledge of food safety control.

REFERENCES

CONNOLLY, A. 1995. National Study of Quality Management Practices in the Irish Food Industry. Report from Centre for Quality and Services Management, Graduate School of Business, University College Dublin, pp. 35.

DALY, P. 1998. Food safety and quality assurance systems at farm level. In *Food Safety: The Implications of Change — From Producerism to Consumerism*, (J.J. Sheridan, M. O'Keeffe and M. Rogers, eds.) Food & Nutrition Press, Trumbull, pp. 197–202.

CHAPTER 16

FOOD SAFETY AND QUALITY ASSURANCE SYSTEMS AT FARM LEVEL

PAT DALY

Teagasc, The National Food Centre
Dunsinea, Castleknock
Dublin 15, Ireland

ABSTRACT

Outbreaks of foodborne illnesses, some with tragic consequences, have raised widespread concern about the ability of the agri food industry to produce safe food. There is increasing acceptance of the food chain concept, whereby practices at any stage in the chain from production to consumption, can impinge on the safety of the final food. In response to both commercial and regulatory pressures, farmers, food processors and retailers are developing and implementing recognised food safety and quality management systems. HACCP (Hazard Analysis Critical Control Point) systems and ISO 9000 standards are internationally recognised model systems for food safety and quality management. These standards, or codes of practice based on them, can be applied to all food production operations, to ensure safe produce at the key first step in the food chain.

An increasing number of intensive farm producers have implemented safety/quality management systems, which has shown that these systems can be successfully applied at farm level. There is a need to extend this approach to all farms producing food. All farmers, intensive or otherwise, must meet current standards in terms of product safety and quality. Producer codes of practice are now available for many farm sectors and used in partnership with food processors provide a system that can be used by all food producers to ensure a safe and quality product for consumers.

INTRODUCTION

This paper outlines how food safety and quality management systems can be applied to farm or primary food production operations. To gain customer acceptance it is important that management systems are based on recognised standards. Internationally recognised food safety and quality management system model standards are available. These are HACCP (Hazard Analysis Critical

Control Point system) and ISO 9000 Quality Systems series of standards which have been in use in the food processing industry for some time. Given the ongoing concerns with food safety and the integrated nature of the food chain, these systems could be applied along the entire food chain. Production codes of practice based on HACCP and ISO 9000 standards are being developed for the various sectors and these standards are being successfully applied at farm level. This should help in reducing incidents of food safety scares and should give increased assurance to the consumer in the safety and quality of foods produced.

BACKGROUND

Quality management systems have been in use since the 1950s. They have their origins in the engineering based defence industries as part of contractual specifications for the purpose of ensuring that products were manufactured to contract. These standards were subsequently adopted across many sectors of manufacturing industry and also as national and international quality management standards.

The HACCP system was used as a means of producing a safe food for the early manned space programmes in the 1960s and 1970s. Commercial applications followed, such as in the production of low acid canned foods. In the subsequent decades HACCP systems have been applied to many food processing industries through regulatory requirements and industry codes of practice.

Recently food safety scares have unfortunately become more prominent, some with tragic consequences. These have sometimes been associated with primary production, for example BSE and *E.coli* O157:H7. While formalised management systems have been in place in the food processing industry for at least ten years, processors are required to have a HACCP system in place. The first principle of HACCP requires that hazards are identified at all stages in the production process. This has fuelled commercial interests and regulatory bodies to focus more closely on controls along the entire food chain, rather than just on food processing operations. There is now an acceptance that adverse practices at any stage of the food chain can impinge on the safety of the final product, the chain being as strong as its weakest link. The adoption of management systems represents a move from external controls on product safety by customers or regulators to the use of self check systems by the producer.

FARM PRACTICES — PRODUCT SAFETY AND QUALITY MANAGEMENT

In relation to the application of management systems at farm level, producers can be divided into three categories, (1) industry type primary producers, such as pig and poultry operations; (2) intensive farm operations, and (3) extensive farming.

However, all primary producers are producing a food either directly for consumption, such as vegetables, or for further processing, irrespective of the size of the operation and all must maintain a minimum standard in relation to food safety. This parallels the food processing industry, where minimum product safety standards must be attained irrespective of company size.

There has already been substantial progress in the uptake of these management systems in primary production. Pig and poultry producers have registered to the ISO 9002 standard. Beef, grain and horticulture quality assurance schemes are in operation. Dairy co-operatives have developed in house codes of practice for their milk suppliers.

Farming Under a Management System

Farm systems can be treated as consisting of: (1) Inputs, (2) Processes and (3) Outputs.

1. Inputs are many and varied. Examples are fertilisers, agrochemicals, seed, feed, and medication. All have the potential to contribute hazards to the final product unless used in a controlled manner.

2. The process involves the various crop or livestock husbandry practices. These include feeding, cleaning, milking, harvesting, storage, and transport. These processes are supported by different checks on the product during production. There are many occasions during the production process where contamination can occur. The use of feed stuffs and in particular medicated feeds creates potential hazards. Possible hazards arise from the mixing of medicated and nonmedicated feeds. The cleaning of storage bins and associated feed lines is critical to avoidance of cross contamination. Identification of animals on medicated feed is necessary. It is possible to observe withdrawal periods if it is known with certainty which batch of animals were given the medicated feed. In milk production, the health or medication status of each cow is vital to ensure a batch of milk is not contaminated. Milking equipment requires proper cleaning to prevent carryover of cleaning agent residues to the milk. The hygiene practices of the milker are important, as they are a potential vehicle for cross contamination between cow and milk. This requires the use of protective clothing and adherence to good hygiene practices, such as regular hand washing. Changes in regulations with legal and voluntary bans on particular feed ingredients further complicates the issue.

Traceability. Traceability is a key part of process control and the focus of much current discussion and research. For large animals, such as cattle it is possible, through tagging, to have some degree of traceability, at least up to primary processing. But for foods such as grain and milk traceability is more difficult because there is mixing from an early stage of production. This difficulty in meeting blanket traceability for foods, as perceived by consumers and often promoted by retailers, further highlights the need for a preventive approach to controlling hazard in foods.

3. Outputs are milk, grain, meat (livestock), vegetables. The safety and quality of produce is dependent on correct storage and transport to the customer.

Product Controls

Demonstrating that best practice exists in producing and handling the various products requires good practices of hygiene and disease control and proper maintenance of records. Controls, such as having a locked medicine cabinet, a secure site, up to date medication and animal identification records. Site security equates to product security and also helps control spread of disease. Other relatively inexpensive but necessary controls are bird exclusion and clear identification of feed bins at grain stores.

Farm Audits

On farm audits are now becoming common practice. These audits usually cover the following areas.

1. **stockmanship**; competence of farm personnel
2. **stock source**; traceability records
3. **animal welfare**; food, water, housing, disease control, stocking rates, isolation facilities, alarm and fail safe systems
4. **herd health**; hygiene standards, disease control, pest control,
5. **feed**; ingredient traceability, diet balance, feed storage, bin/line cleaning
6. **medications**; storage, usage, withdrawal periods, administration procedure, application level

Audits give an indication of the topics that codes of practice at farm level need to address. A typical code of practice for milk production would include, animal health and welfare, stockmanship, nutrition, milking practices, milk quality standards and waste management. These headings would be applicable to any producers code of practice with the inclusion of the appropriate product standard and transport for livestock. Animal welfare and waste management are now standard inclusions in producer codes of practice, as the consumer is becoming increasingly concerned about where the food comes from and what damage, if any, is being done to the environment.

SYSTEM IMPLEMENTATION

There is a recognised approach to developing a safety quality management system. This requires input from the experts in the factors affecting the safety and quality of the produce. In practice this includes, animal health, animal husbandry, nutrition specialists and a knowledge of customer and regulatory requirements. Acceptable levels have to be established for identified hazards such as agrochemical, antibiotic residues and pathogens. Codes of practice are now rapidly being produced for the various sectors but having the code is only the start. All producers must implement the codes. Implementation demands resources in terms of time and energy.

Implementing systems requires both education and training. Education is required to convince producers of the need for maintaining systems and understanding customer requirements. Training is required to ensure that people understand and can follow procedures on a consistent basis. This might be the correct application of agrochemicals, medication, equipment cleaning and completion of records. Training is also necessary to ensure that personnel present themselves and the enterprise to the optimum during a customer audit. Increasingly customers need external verification that personnel have been trained in safe food production practices, such as certificates of attendance at approved courses.

Traditionally, processors were in the happy position of being able to nominate to their customers — often the retail supermarkets — the supplier that should be visited. Obviously, this could be the particular award winning supplier. That is no longer the case. The customers want to look at the supplier list and make the selection themselves.

It is important to recognise that all standards are updated to reflect changing requirements which generally means becoming more stringent. Systems will manage known hazards but the ability to recognise and control emerging hazards need to be incorporated into the control system. In this respect continuous research is vital on new or emerging hazards and their control. Specific examples of where updates have taken place are the inclusion of equipment maintenance in the ISO 9002 standard. This has relevance in farming, for example, the maintenance of milking machines, grain dryers and temperature/ventilation control in pig or poultry operations.

The maintenance of records is important in management systems as a means of demonstrating consistent control of the process. Examples in the use of agrochemicals are application rate, type, when/were applied and when product was harvested.

CONCLUSION

Farmers have shown the ability to adapt to change in the marketplace. Examples include new technologies, scale of operations, animal breeds, crop varieties and production quota systems. They have the benefit of the experience of the process industries where food safety and quality management systems have been in place for many years and in many cases have established links with these processors through supplier contracts.

The HACCP system and ISO 9000 Standards provide a suitable model and a systematic approach to developing a food safety and quality management system at primary production level. These systems are based on preventing problems and are internationally recognised, hence offer the potential for better use of available resources, and for customer acceptance. The systems can be applied at all stages in the food chain giving a uniform approach to ensuring the safety and quality of food. The existence of a formal documented system will increase awareness on the part of the producer of production factors that affect the safety and quality of produce. The existence of verifiable systems will help in giving increased assurance to the consumer of the safety and quality of produce.

CHAPTER 17

ANIMAL TRACEABILITY IN NORTHERN IRELAND AND ITS RELEVANCE TO PRODUCING SAFER FOOD

R.M. McCRACKEN

Veterinary Service
Department of Agriculture for Northern Ireland
Dundonald House
Belfast, BT4 3SB

ABSTRACT

Food is derived from live organisms and the implications of this must be recognised in all programmes geared towards the production of food. Recent food scares emphasise the need for meat inspection to be performed at a consistently high standard. The consumer has every right and every expectation that food purchased in retail outlets should be safe and wholesome. The confidence of the consumer throughout the EU has been shaken by a series of events which include salmonellosis, listeriosis, *drug residues, BSE and* E. coli O157:H7. *The consumer now demands credible assurances and guarantees from an impartial and objective body.*

Such assurances and guarantees must be based on a clear knowledge of both the production and processing stages involved in food production. They must be delivered through a mechanism which monitors individual animals through production and processing. The idea that food production starts only when the animal arrives at the slaughter house is outdated and senseless. Monitoring from "conception to consumption" must be the goal. The Veterinary Service in the Department of Agriculture for Northern Ireland is an holistic service with responsibility and accountability for animal health and welfare and for veterinary public health. Monitoring of the disease status of cattle is effected through a computerised Animal Health System (AHS), as are the unique ear number, movement records, breed, sex, age, and colour of each bovine in Northern Ireland.

This paper describes how the Veterinary Service in Northern Ireland has utilised its centralised AHS computer to deliver meaningful assurances and guarantees and is looking forward to the replacement computerised system, due for implementation within the next twelve months.

INTRODUCTION

Twenty years ago most farmers' aims and concerns centred around being able to sell heavy, fat animals to the abattoir. Meeting the concerns of the consumer was a matter entirely for abattoir management and others. Such an attitude has long since disappeared and the production of animals, their slaughter and processing and the marketing of meat is an holistic activity involving all, from "conception to consumption". The numbers of live animals in Northern Ireland and the slaughterings are shown in Table 1. Today's farmer is concerned with meeting the needs of the consumer and strives to do so. In Northern Ireland and indeed throughout our island, almost 80% of all beef produced is exported. This has helped focus farmers' minds on what is important, meeting the real needs and perceived needs of the consumer, at home and abroad.

TABLE 1.
NUMBER OF ANIMALS AND SLAUGHTERINGS IN NORTHERN IRELAND

Species	Population (millions)	Slaughterings (millions)
Cattle	1.5	0.5
Sheep	2.5	1.0
Pig	1.2	0.6
Poultry	65.0	13.6

Northern Ireland has an advantage over several other member states in that the slaughtering and processing industry is operated through a very small number of modern, well run plants. These plants have all been EU and third world country approved for many years which is a reflection of their dependency on being able to export. The role of government is to ensure that meat is wholesome and safe and that all other players are committed to similar objectives.

The Veterinary Service in Northern Ireland has responsibility and accountability from the birth of calves through to marketing of the beef. In exercising such responsibilities and accountabilities adequate tools are needed. The centralised, computerised system called the Animal Health System (AHS) for cattle is one of several important and vital tools in the successful delivery of this service. The strengths of the veterinary service stem from it being an holistic service, from the good quality healthy stock, from the short distances to abattoirs and from the existence of traceability.

THE ANIMAL HEALTH SYSTEM

Looking back to events prior to 20 March 1996, the Northern Ireland beef industry was exporting products throughout the EU and to many third world countries. Indeed, in one instance a company within another member state was sourcing its beef entirely from Northern Ireland. Given the fact that Northern Ireland was classified as having a "high incidence" of BSE, the question could be asked as to why another country sourced its beef from Northern Ireland. The answer is twofold: the beef is of consistently high quality and both these customers and their consumers had full confidence in the assurances and guarantees provided by industry and by the Department of Agriculture for Northern Ireland. It is most likely that the absence of a computerised traceability system would have made such trade impossible. Through the AHS there exists a dynamic and reactive record of all cattle details, movements and disease testing histories. The AHS was implemented over ten years ago and is centred around the bovine's unique identification number, contained on the ear tag. The details of the information on the ear tag in shown in Table 2.

TABLE 2.
INFORMATION AVAILABLE FROM EAR TAGS ON CATTLE IN NORTHERN IRELAND

Example Number:	654321-1234
Key: 654321	Farmer's Herd Number
1234	Number of Individual Animal
X	Computer Check Digit

In addition to the ear tag number, the computer also contains details on each animal. These include breed, colour, sex, date of birth, disease status including contact with BSE, farm quality assurance status and entire movement records (Table 3).

TABLE 3.
DETAILED DESCRIPTION OF EACH ANIMAL ON COMPUTER SYSTEM

Tag No.	Prev/RoI/PED	OTM	Col	Br	Sex	Birth
06173-1392-R	RWJ 6B	O	BW	DAQ	F	011293

Key: RWJ6B = Previous tag number
O = Over 30 months of age
BW = Black and white in colour
DAQ = Blonde D'Aquitaine breed
F = Female

Based on the ear tag number, the AHS produces a full movement history for all cattle in a herd or for an individual animal within the herd (Table 4).

TABLE 4.
MOVEMENT HISTORY OF ANIMALS SHOWING TRACEABILITY FROM BIRTH TO SLAUGHTER

Surname		McCartan	Herd Number 0499 TA-AMH		
Forename		Joe	Tag 06163-1392-R		
Tag number	Issue Herd	Receiving herd	Date moved	Move Cat	Permit Number
06163-1392-R	06163		010594	B	
06163-1392-R	06163	MO4A18	150594	2	
06163-1392-R	MO4A18	0499	150594	1	
06163-1392-R	0499	A09001	060896	2	011546878C

Key: M = Market
A = Abattoir
B = Base capture date (normally born into a herd or imported)
1 = Permit issued by veterinary service
2 = Farmer's self written declaration
TA-AMH = Trace animal - animal movement history
Permit number = Permit number remains against a herd until the move has been confirmed by a Department of Agriculture test or another move.

All cattle movements in Northern Ireland are effected through permits, issued by the Veterinary Service or based on farmer, self-written permits depending on the type of animal being moved. In this way it is relatively easy to trace an animal from birth through to the abattoir. In so doing, the health status of the animal and every herd in which it has been can be ascertained.

Since the appearance of BSE, and the requirement to identify all cattle that were born in or ever passed through a herd in which a case of BSE has occurred, it has been possible to employ the AHS to carry out this task. Thus, when a case of BSE is confirmed in a herd, all cattle that had been in that herd in the past 6 years are automatically identified and flagged. Likewise, all existing cattle in the herd and all future cattle for the next 6 years are and will be automatically flagged. To provide such a service by the manual route is unwieldy and fraught with problems; computerised records make it an easy task. As only meat from cattle of less than 30 months of age can be sold for human consumption, AHS has been programmed whereby a marker indicates whether each bovine is less than 30 or greater than 30 months of age. This is reassessed on a daily basis. Additionally, cattle are flagged as meeting or not meeting Farm Quality Assured criteria (Table 5).

TABLE 5.
THE BSE HERD LIST DISPLAYING THE BSE STATUS, QUALITY AND AGE OF ANIMALS

Herd (1234)	Name		(Joe Smith)	Tel (0266 65163)
Area (3J)			(Main Street)	PVP (s) (MO3)
Herd restrictions	High tag range		(Armagh)	
Tags in herd (10)	(0250)			
			BSE (Y/N)	

Tag number		BF	QL	MF
0499- 43-B		X		O
1234-146-E		-	Q	M
0499-142-A		X		O
3375463PQR UK	I	X		O
391-7393-R		Z		O

Key:
- X = Animal over 30 months of age from BSE herd
- Z = Unrestricted animal after 8 years (Decision 98/256) i.e. animal which was present in a BSE herd during 8 year restriction period
- Q = Quality assured animal
- O = More than 30 months
- M = Less than 30 months
- PVP = Herd owner's private veterinary practitioner
- MO3 = User code for PVP
- BSE (Yes/No) = is the herd subject to BSE restrictions
- BF = BSE flag
- QL = Quality assurance indicator
- MF = Animal age indicator
- I = Animal imported from Great Britain, treated as if it came from a BSE herd

Imported cattle from Great Britain automatically get a BSE flag. Whilst they may be from a non-BSE herd when purchased, the herd of birth and rearing in Great Britain could develop a case of BSE subsequent to importation of the animal to Northern Ireland and this would not be known. However, where necessary, the status of the relevant herds in Great Britain can be ascertained at time of slaughter and the BSE status adjusted accordingly. Cattle imported from other member states or third world countries are also identified on the AHS by a specific country identifier (Table 6).

To assist the Veterinary Service in this work, networked, computer terminals are situated in all Divisional Veterinary Offices, all red meat abattoirs, at rendering plants, ports and at all major cattle markets.

Prior to 20 March 1996, Northern Ireland was marketing beef within the EU and to many third world countries. This trade existed even though BSE was present in Northern Ireland and is an indication of the confidence which importers placed in the traceability system and the assurances it provided. Following the announcements on 20 March 1996 on possible links between BSE and the new variant form of Creutzfeldt-Jakob disease (nvCJD) these markets were lost for all of the UK beef industry.

TABLE 6.
BSE STATUS, POSSIBLE CONTACTS WITH OTHER BSE ANIMALS AND IMPORT DATA FOR ANIMALS PRESENTED FOR SLAUGHTER

Kill date	Kill number	Tag number	Permit number	BSE	Import
300995	3787	06163-1392-R	096546878C	X	
300995	3756	39203-4294-Z	041284572L	Y	
300995	3783	6121319-1848	041284505N	I	UK
300995	3784	63694-5-SAB	041284505N	W	IE
300995	3785	59395-2384-Y	041284505N	X	
300995	3786	49271-4123-Y	034128450H	Z	
080995	3410	54257-6-EJA	C233619	-	IE
080995	3411	77766-9-EIA	C233619	-	IE

Key: I = Animal imported from Great Britain, treated as if it came from a BSE herd
W = Animal less than 30 months of age from a BSE herd
X = Animal over 30 months of age from a BSE herd
Y = Animal born or moved into a herd which was BSE restricted but not restricted now
Z = Unrestricted after 8 years
IE = Republic of Ireland

Since its first appearance in Northern Ireland in November 1988, 1762 BSE cases had been confirmed by the end of October 1997 (Fig. 1). The monthly totals peaked in 1993 and, since then, have shown a steady and predictable decline. The decline is due to the control measures introduced throughout the UK, especially the ban on the use of meat and bone meal in ruminant feeds.

In January 1992 it was predicted in Northern Ireland that the disease would peak in 1993 and reach close to sporadic occurrence before the end of the century. It is encouraging to note that the actual incidences experienced are very similar to those predicted.

The significance of the AHS computer at abattoir level is considerable. The system is live and dynamic and veterinary checks are made before the animals are off-loaded, using the permits which accompany the cattle to the abattoir. If animals are not eligible for entry into the abattoir they are penned and slaughtered separately, depending on criteria such as BSE and Farm Quality Assured status. In order to ensure that meat can be traced back, not only to the abattoir but to the farms of birth, rearing and finishing, the kill number is correlated with the unique identification number (ear tag number) of the live animal and the Bar Code Number generated in the abattoir and used on the packages of beef.

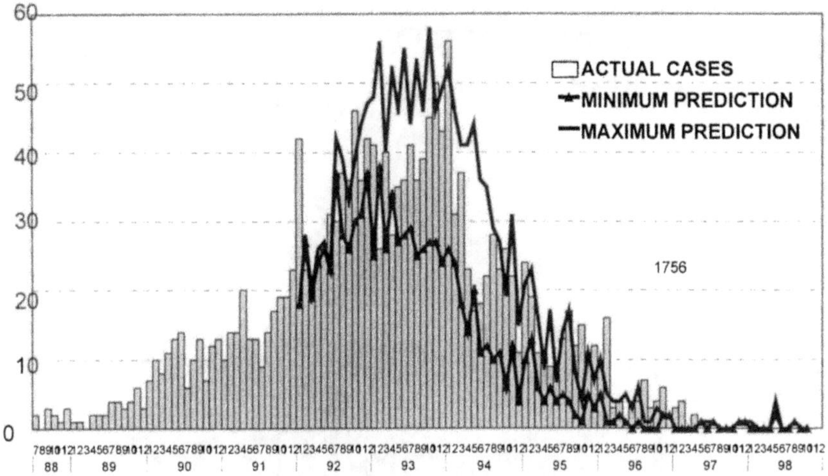

FIG. 1. ACTUAL AND PREDICTED CASES OF BSE FROM 1992 ONWARDS IN NORTHERN IRELAND. CASES BY MONTH OF CLINICAL ONSET.

When the system moves to a new computer, an improved efficiency is planned in relation to the linkage between the live animal and the beef sold in retail outlets. Furthermore, some supermarket operators, at home and abroad are now seeking beef from cattle which have only been on one or two farms. The movement recording system allows the identification of animals which qualify for such trade. Undoubtedly, the consumer and the large supermarket chains will require other criteria to be met and it is certain that a computerised system is generally best placed to provide the assurances sought.

CONCLUSION

The AHS, and the updated version which becomes operational from mid-1998, will continue to be an essential tool in providing the food industry and its consumers with the necessary assurances and guarantees. It is difficult to imagine how such high level quality assurances could be provided without computerisation. A partial lifting of the export ban on UK beef is anticipated and, with the help of the present traceability system, the beef industry will then be in a position to win back markets through the quality of the assurances the computerised traceability system can help to provide.

CHAPTER 18

THE DEVELOPMENT OF AN ANIMAL TRACEABILITY SYSTEM FOR USE IN FOOD SAFETY ASSURANCE SCHEMES

TOM ARNOLD

Department of Agriculture and Food
Kildare St., Dublin 2
Ireland

ABSTRACT

In May 1997, the National Beef Assurance Scheme (NBAS) was launched by the Minister for Agriculture and Food, Mr. Ivan Yates, TD. Under the NBAS, the Department of Agriculture and Food will introduce arrangements on standards to be applied and observed under a registration system by farmers, meat processors, marts and feed compounders. The system will have independent inspection and monitoring. A further major commitment in the NBAS is the introduction of a Computerised Movement System (CMMS). This paper provides a description of what is involved under the CMMS and an update on the progress in its implementation. CMMS will, when fully operational, provide a computerised bovine animal traceability file. Apart from the commitment made in NBAS to establish CMMS, there is, in any event, a mandatory requirement on the Department, under recently adopted European Union legislation, to put in place a comprehensive computerised animal traceability system by the end of 1999. Failure to do so will jeopardise Ireland's ability to trade animals and animal products and could also have implications for receipts under the various headage and premium schemes. The Department has already developed an Animal Location File (ALF), which contains data on an animal's location at specific points during its lifetime (headage and premium schemes, export plants and ports, etc.). Developing the CMMS will require collection of data at a whole range of new locations, e.g. marts and inter-farm movements. The project represents a considerable challenge in organisational and information technology (IT) terms. The organisational challenge is in terms of the arrangements which have to be agreed between the Department and a significant number of agencies (e.g. farm organisations, marts, meat factories). The IT challenge is in terms of the design of the system to capture and process the data on animal movements, such that CMMS can be effectively used as an instrument to clear animals into the food chain (domestic and foreign) and for live export.

INTRODUCTION

Before dealing with the assurance schemes and the traceability arrangements which are the subject of this paper, it is important to place the Irish beef industry into its economic context. About 150,000 herd owners are engaged in cattle production, the output value of which was IR£1150m in 1996. Some 5,000 people are employed in beef processing. The value of cattle and beef exports, taking account of the associated export refunds, amounted to just over IR£1 billion in 1996. In short, the beef industry is of vital importance to the national economy and needs to be underpinned by whatever administrative and regulatory arrangements are necessary to ensure its capacity to trade.

The obligations which this country must meet in its trading arrangements with other countries became more stringent from March 1996, following the British Government announcement of a link between BSE and a new variant of CJD in young people. The export of British beef was banned within the European Union (EU) and to third world countries. The knock-on effect was a substantial reduction in beef consumption within the EU — which has recovered somewhat in the past year. In addition, a number of markets to which Ireland supplied cattle and beef products imposed full or partial trade restrictions on Irish cattle and beef exports.

The key response to this situation at EU and national level has been to seek to provide assurance to domestic and foreign consumers and markets as to the safety of cattle and beef products.

European Union (EU)

At EU level there has been a broad based response to food safety. From the perspective of the Irish Department of Agriculture and Food, the major components of this response have been:

1. A new political departure in the fields of scientific advice, risk analysis and control and inspection put forward by the Commission in its communication on consumer health and food safety. This approach is based on a separation of responsibilities for legislation on the one hand and for scientific advice, control and inspection on the other. It has been translated into a major reorganisation of Commission services which should ensure that the Commission is in a position to react appropriately to the challenges in the field of consumer health.
2. A green paper on food law has been issued. Consultations have just ended, including a major contribution from consumer associations. A proposal for a draft Directive on an extension of product liability to include primary agricultural products has been decided upon by the Commission.

3. Article 129 of the Amsterdam Treaty provides a new legal basis for co-decision between the European Parliament and the Council on veterinary and phyto-sanitary matters directly related to public health protection. Consumer policy in general is strengthened by the revised Article 129a.
4. The Agenda 2000 proposals contain major reforms of the Common Agriculture Policy (CAP) directed towards sustainable farming and the production of safe and healthy food.
5. Specifically in relation to animal traceability, a Council Regulation No. 820/97 on animal identification, registration and traceability was agreed and applied from 1 July 1997. Among the requirements of this Regulation are:

   (a) A standard EU system of eartag identification to operate from 1 January 1998 for animals born after that date.
   (b) The requirements on all keepers of animals to complete an Animal Identification Document (called a "passport") recording each movement onto or off holdings.
   (c) As an alternative to the latter, the requirement on all keepers of animals to notify all movements onto or off holdings to the competent authority of the Member State in the context of the competent authority having an operational database to record all traceability events (such as births, movements, disposals). All Member States are required to have such a traceability database in place not later than 31 December 1999.

National

At national level, the Government took a number of measures to address immediate and long term issues, in particular:

1. It strengthened controls at its borders and introduced measures to safeguard public and animal health and to combat BSE.
2. It developed an Animal Location File (ALF) and introduced a movement permit system for female cattle entering meat plants and being exported.
3. It decided to establish the Food Safety Authority of Ireland which will have responsibility for food safety and hygiene.

It developed a National Beef Assurance Scheme (NBAS), the outline of which was announced in May 1997, and the principal elements of which are:

(a) A Computerised Movement Monitoring System (CMMS)
(b) Farm and Factory Protocols
(c) Feedingstuffs and Marts protocols

COMPUTERISED MOVEMENT MONITORING SYSTEM (CMMS)

The CMMS involves the establishment of a fully computerised system for the identification of cattle and for the monitoring of all cattle movements. This paper outlines what its principal components are, what progress has been made in its implementation and what remains to be done. The fundamental objective of the CMMS is to create a computerised bovine animal traceability file. It aims to put in place the arrangements necessary to enable data on animal movements (farm to farm, farm to mart, mart to farm, etc.) to be recorded and to create the computer facilities for receiving and storing this data. This database can then be used to validate the origins and locations of animals at time of slaughter or export.

The development of the CMMS database will build on the existing Animal Location File (ALF) database. This database was developed during 1996 in response to the need for assurance for domestic consumers and export markets. It brought together data from the existing systems/schemes operated by the Department of Agriculture and Food, such as the Calf Registration system and the Headage and Premium schemes. It also included data on slaughtering at export plants and live exports. What ALF did not have was data on animal movements between these locations.

Data for CMMS

CMMS will be a centrally located, controlled and managed computer facility. Every individual animal movement will have to be notified to the central agency by the parties involved; this will include farmers, dealers, agents, marts, export factories, abattoirs, live export points and others. The data to be entered on CMMS will deal with movements which have occurred.

Marts will have a key role in capturing data on cattle movement, given that the bulk of cattle movements in Ireland pass through them. Marts will record the identity of animals being traded and the source herd and herd of destination. The mart will pass that data to CMMS. For that purpose it is intended to use to the maximum extent possible direct computer links between the marts and the Department of Agriculture and Food's central computer on which CMMS is stored. In this regard the Department intends providing the necessary communication links and PCs to the marts. Data on inter-farm movement (farmers, dealer, agent) will involve notifications to be completed by both the buyer and seller of the cattle. These notifications will be fed to the central database either through the District Veterinary Offices (DVOs) or to a central data capture agency acting on behalf of the Department of Agriculture and Food. For end of line locations, such as export factories, large abattoirs and live export points, computer facilities will be provided to facilitate the validation of cattle presented and to pass on the identity of the animals and their herds of origin to the central system.

Links With Other Departmental Computer Systems

The development and design of the CMMS will take account of the need to integrate and pass data between the major departmental systems. Redesign and redevelopment of the current Disease Testing system will commence during 1998 and its data will be integrated into the CMMS. Further attention will be given to providing linkages between the CMMS database and the database which currently runs the Headage and Premium schemes and with other herd based information.

Organisational and Legislative Aspects of CMMS

Department of Agriculture and Food. The implementation of CMMS is a major organisational challenge, to the Department of Agriculture and Food and to the farming and cattle trading sector. Within the Department, overall responsibility for CMMS implementation has been given to a newly created division dealing with the NBAS. This division will be required to liase with a number of administrative and veterinary Divisions with various executive responsibilities in CMMS implementation, and in particular with the Department's Information System (Computer) Division. The division will also be responsible for the execution and management of a National Herd Census, as well as an effective Monitoring/Policing/Penalty Unit which will have to be in place to ensure compliance with the animal movement notification arrangements to be operated by farmers and others.

Legislative. The division will also be responsible for ensuring that there is an appropriate legislative basis for the operation of the overall NBAS, including CMMS. EU legislation on animal identification and registration systems and on trading in animals, along with national legislation on animal health, disease prevention, export and marts, give a solid foundation, but additional primary and secondary legislation is likely to be necessary.

As already mentioned, Council Regulation No. 820/97 currently sets out the EU legal requirements in relation to animal identification, registration and traceability. In addition to this, Commission proposals for the detailed operational aspects are being finalised at working group level in Brussels. These will provide for a whole range of measures including the levels of controls to be carried out, together with a series of penalties that can be applied by member states where breaches of the identification and movement requirements are detected. Examples of current Commission thinking on penalisation include:

1. Restrictions on the movement of the animals to or from the holdings concerned, in cases where there are unidentified animals or animals for which the identification and registration requirements are not fully met;
2. Any animal that cannot be identified within 24 hours should be slaughtered without compensation;
3. Where the number of incorrectly identified or incorrectly registered animals on a holding is in excess of 10%, all the animals present on the holding should be slaughtered without compensation;
4. Farmers should be excluded wholly or partially from support arrangements under the CAP;
5. Criminal penalties, depending on the seriousness of the infringement identified.

Farmer and Trading Sector. Implementation of CMMS will also have major organisational implications for the Department of Agriculture and Food, farmers and the cattle trading system. The gathering of the animal data will require a whole range of new actions and activities, on the part of Department of Agriculture and Food staff either directly or in checking, monitoring and controlling the actions of others, e.g.

1. at Marts (about 130)
2. at Meat Factories (about 30)
3. at Abattoirs (about 450)
4. at Ports and live animal Assembly Points (6-10)
5. by Farmers (many thousands involved in inter-herd transfers)
6. a national Herd Census (about 150,000 herds)

The precise nature of the tasks involved in data collection and transmission, and the respective responsibilities between Department of Agriculture and Food staff and marts, factories, etc. are being worked out through a process of consultation. A number of pilot projects have been initiated with marts to assess the most effective means of implementing the CMMS. Similar exercises will be undertaken at meat factories and abattoirs as soon as possible. It is envisaged that Departmental staff will undertake the activities at export points.

Financing of the CMMS

A considerable investment has already been made towards the establishment of the CMMS. In 1997, some IR£4m was provided for NBAS/CMMS activities. This has covered the enhancement of central computer facilities and increased capacity; the provision of appropriate computer facilities and links at the various locations (marts, factories, etc.) both for data input and for database enquiry access; the design and development of the computer system on which the data will be stored; the use of data capture facilities, and consultancy costs and systems design. Funding for NBAS/CMMS in 1998 will allow for commencement of the redesign of the Disease Testing System, from which the herd data will be integrated into the CMMS.

Timing of Implementation

Due to delays in finalising the rules at EU level, resource constraints at Departmental and other areas, and the scale of the organisational tasks which CMMS represents, there has been some slippage in the dates for CMMS implementation which were announced in May 1997 as part of the NBAS. Piloting of the system in marts is commencing towards the end of 1997 and other pilots will follow. The other main 'next steps' to be implemented relate to gathering slaughter and disposal data on animals; the introduction of a farmer animal movement notification system, and finally the holding of a national herd census.

Use of CMMS in Assurance Schemes

All parties recognise the vital contribution which a proper identification and movement monitoring system can make to reassuring consumers both at home and abroad. However, the implications and the disciplines that will be required of a range of parties under a fully operational system may not be fully appreciated by everybody. The scale of the operational aspects and the information that will have to be assembled, co-ordinated and monitored has been outlined briefly above. This information will ultimately be used to validate the life history of each animal before it enters the food chain or is exported. This is an important aspect but it is sometimes not fully appreciated and will have major implications for final producers in particular; it is however an indispensable element of any assurance scheme. Other elements of the beef assurance scheme include;

(a) rigorous residue testing procedures for illegal or undesirable substances.
(b) effective monitoring of factory conditions, processes and procedures.

The finalisation of the details of all of these arrangements is continuing with a view to introduction of the beef assurance scheme in 1998.

CHAPTER 19

CONTROLLED QUALITY MEAT: THE DUTCH EXPERIENCE

HENK BEKMAN

Product Boards for Livestock, Meat and Eggs
Sir Winston Churchilllaan 275, Postbus 5805
2280 HV, Rijswijk, The Netherlands

ABSTRACT

During the last few years there is a growing feeling in the Dutch livestock and meat industry that it is essential to change from a product oriented to a more market-oriented production (from quantity to quality). This is mainly due to developments such as a more intense international competition, stagnant or declining meat consumption and negative pressure on the consumers' image of meat. Counteracting these developments is only possible if every part of the production chain contributes (in close cooperation with each other) to achieve a better control of the whole production process: from conception to consumption. For a number of years an extensive research programme has been carried out to set up a system of Integrated Quality Control (IKB). This has led to a "total quality concept" which includes the safety and quality of the product, the production method, care for the environment, and human and animal health. This paper discusses the basic elements (structure and content) of this quality concept. The extent of implementation of the IKB-concept depends on the particular sector, but it is at around 70% for pigs and broilers. For IKB in veal, current participation is over 90%.

INTRODUCTION

The livestock and meat industry (including poultry and eggs) is very important for the Dutch economy. In 1996 1.2 million cattle, 1.2 million calves, almost 18.5 million pigs and 400 million poultry were slaughtered in the Netherlands. Furthermore 9.0 billion eggs were produced. Of the total production in this sector, 70% was exported with a value (in 1996) of approximately 12.5 billion Dutch guilders (PVV 1997). This is a result of an impressive growth in production during the last two decades.

During the last few years, however, there is a growing feeling in our industry that it is necessary to change from a production driven to a more consumer and market-oriented system: **from quantity to quality**. This is mainly due to developments such as: (1) more intensified international competition; (2) stagnation or decline in meat consumption in our traditional markets; (3) increased costs and lower prices (GATT, environment), and (4) negative pressure on the consumers' image of meat.

In many countries, especially in Europe and North America, there is a growing concern among consumers about the origin, safety and wholesomeness of their daily food in general and of meat in particular. Therefore, consumers are demanding more guarantees with regard to the quality and safety of meat.

Consumer research in the Netherlands has confirmed that the consumers' image of meat production is influenced negatively in relation to these aspects (Candel *et al.* 1998). In the long run this can be expected to have a negative effect on meat consumption.

Solution to the Problem

The first concern is to produce what the consumer wants. Secondly, and more importantly, it is to give better guarantees that the quality of the product is what was promised. These are easy statements to make, but difficult to put into consistent practice.

In the 1980's the first discussions on this topic started. It was recognised by the industry that the quality and wholesomeness of meat is influenced by all parts of the production chain. Therefore only an integrated, i.e. one covering the whole production chain, would be successful, an approach whereby all parts of the chain have to be involved in close cooperation. The primary responsibility for the quality and safety of the product must lie with the producer. The role of the government should be restricted to that of a supervisor for those aspects relating to public health. This philosophy now is known in the Dutch meat industry under the term IKB (Integrale Keten Beheersing or Integrated Chain Control).

THE IKB APPROACH IN THE NETHERLANDS

IKB means a Quality Assurance System (QAS) approach for the whole production chain. In this respect it is important to stress that IKB, being a quality assurance system, is not a goal in itself, but is "merely" an infrastructure (the railway) to guarantee that the product meets certain minimal quality requirements (e.g. the train on the railway). The particular requirements which need to be fulfilled depend on the demands of the market and/or the quality goals of the company itself. Besides that, the primary goal of IKB is not improvement of the product quality itself (in the Netherlands this was and is already at a high level), but improvement of the guarantee that a product of good quality is being produced.

In the Netherlands there are IKB-schemes for veal calves, pigs, broilers, eggs, turkey and cattle. Important elements of every IKB-scheme are: (1) one national scheme per species with uniform minimum requirements, (2) participation on a voluntary basis, (3) participation being open to foreign companies, (4) the scheme applies to the whole production chain, (5) traceability of animals, meat and eggs is guaranteed, (6) internal inspection organizations are STERIN-qualified (i.e. certified/accredited to international standards EN 45004), (7) audits and sanctions by an independent organisation, (8) recording and exchange of relevant information between different parts of the production chain, and (9) the system is specified/described in quality manuals. All IKB-schemes are set up in close cooperation between the product board and the industry. The different IKB-programmes already contain a great number of elements of ISO-9000 standards for QAS-systems. The product quality requirements depend on the market and differ between the IKB-schemes. In the schemes for veal and beef there is the guarantee that no growth promotors are used. For poultry and eggs the central point is the microbiological quality, while for pigs it is the correct use of veterinary drugs and absence of residues.

Furthermore, IKB has stimulated companies to give more attention to quality assurance systems in other parts of their operation, e.g. HACCP, environmental aspects, employee-working conditions. More and more companies are receiving ISO-9000 certificates for their IKB-systems. These initiatives show that thinking and acting according to IKB-principles is spreading rapidly through the Dutch livestock and meat industry.

OVERVIEW OF THE DIFFERENT IKB-SCHEMES IN THE NETHERLANDS

IKB Pigs

The IKB-scheme for pigs started in 1992. The most important product regulations in the scheme relate to the traceability, feed quality, hygiene, use of veterinary drugs and (absence of) residues.

The slaughterhouse plays a central role in creating an IKB-production chain for the primary production. The slaughterhouse must develop a quality assurance system for the production chain and this must be specified/described in a manual. The system is then audited on behalf of the Product Board by an audit team from the TNO and SGS-Agrocontrol organisations. Only after a positive judgement by the auditors does the slaughterhouse (and therefore the whole production chain) get the IKB-certificate.

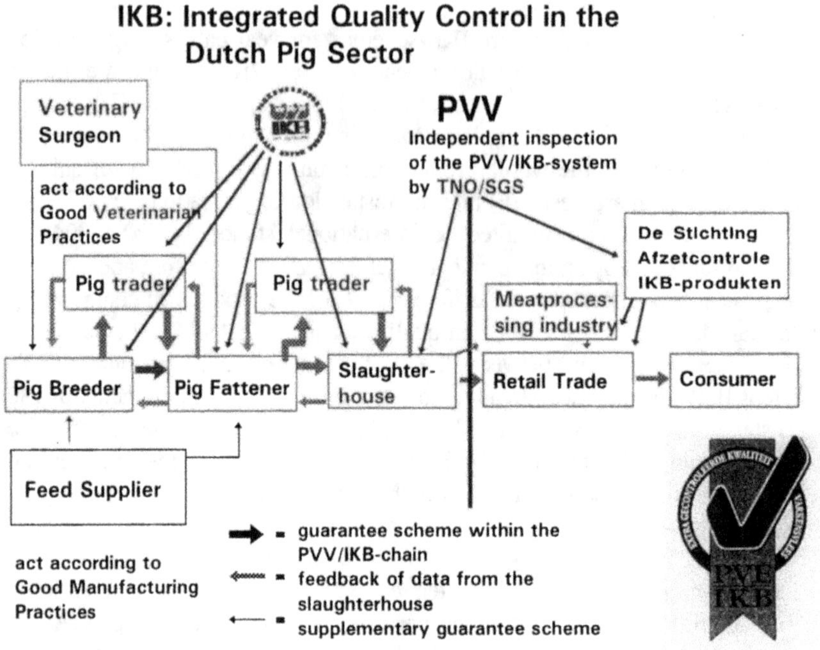

FIG. 1. THE SCHEME COVERS THE PRODUCTION CHAIN FROM THE BREEDER UP TO THE RETAILER

An essential part of the whole scheme is a system of independent audits and sanctions. These consist of: (1) internal audit of all participants in a chain twice-a-year, to be carried out by the STERIN-qualified veterinary service inspections unit, (2) an external audit of the quality assurance system of the slaughterhouse twice-a-year on behalf of the Product Board, and (3) if necessary sanctions are applied, and these vary from a warning and/or additional inspection to exclusion from the scheme during a certain period. Not only must the participants in the pig production chain comply with certain rules, but their suppliers, i.e. the feed industry, veterinary surgeons, etc. also have to comply with similar certified quality assurance schemes, set up by their own organisations.

Present situation. The number of participants has grown very rapidly during the last three years (Fig. 2). Presently there are 10,000 farmers with IKB-certificates who produce around 13.5 million pigs per year (75% of Dutch production). All major pig-slaughterhouses have an IKB-certificate (97% of total slaughter capacity).

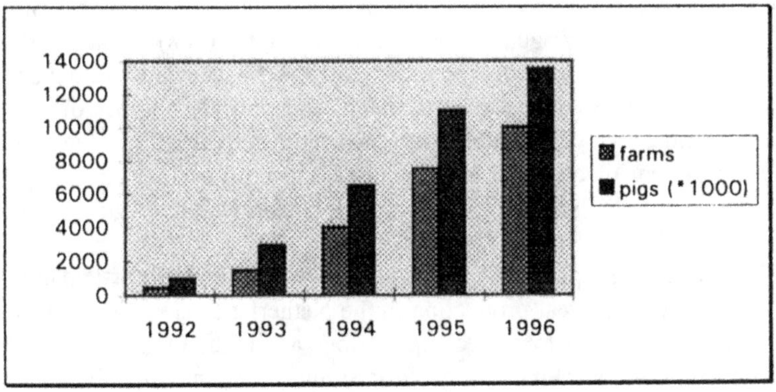

FIG. 2. IKB-PARTICIPATION IN NUMBER OF FARMS AND PIGS

In Holland, retailers, both supermarket chains as well as local butchers, and their customers are interested in the scheme: the pork produced according to the IKB-scheme is already widely considered as the standard product. Most supermarket chains in Holland only buy pork from IKB-certified suppliers. The same developments can be seen in Dutch export markets.

IKB and the Consumer. An important goal of IKB is to improve the consumers' image of meat. Results from recent consumer research indicate that the consumer image of "IKB-pork" is definitely better than the image of "standard pork". The improvement is especially concerned with the weak points of the image of meat, e.g. safety and wholesomeness. There is even an improvement in the image aspects such as animal welfare, tenderness and sensory quality.

On the basis of these results and the availability of the product, by the end of 1995 the scheme will also be open for participation by the retailer. At the same time a consumer logo for IKB-pork has been developed, so that IKB-pork is already visible to the Dutch consumer in the shop. Today there are about 1,350 accredited retail outlets altogether where IKB-pork is on sale.

If this initiative has positive results, there are plans to use the logo for other products like veal and beef and perhaps poultry and eggs.

IKB Veal Calves (SKV)

The IKB-scheme in the veal calf sector is better known as SKV (Foundation for the Quality Guarantee in the Veal Sector). This scheme started in 1991 and is being financed (as are all IKB-schemes) by the industry itself. The most important goal is to give guarantees with regard to the (non) use and absence in the meat of prohibited growth promotors. In 1997 the scheme was extended with regulations relating to the use of veterinary drugs and (the absence of) residues. To achieve this, a very strict and costly (approximately 4 million Dutch guilders per year) system of controls and sanctions has been set up. An independent organization runs the scheme and checks are performed on a regular basis at all parts of the veal production chain.

This scheme has proven to be very successful. Although participation is on a voluntary basis, all veal production in the Netherlands is by this scheme. The meat can be recognized by a special SKV-logo and in the future probably by the IKB-logo. The scheme has also given customers at home and abroad a much greater confidence in the quality of the product.

IKB Broilers

This program started in 1992. The most important element here is improvement in the microbiological quality (e.g. *Salmonella*) of the product. In 1997 the scheme was upgraded with the introduction of an intense scheme of analyses of the *Salmonella*-status in all phases of production. Samples are taken from incoming and outgoing elements of the production. At present around 70% of the national broiler production is in the scheme (see Fig. 3). In total about 2,000 farms are participating in the scheme (PPE 1997).

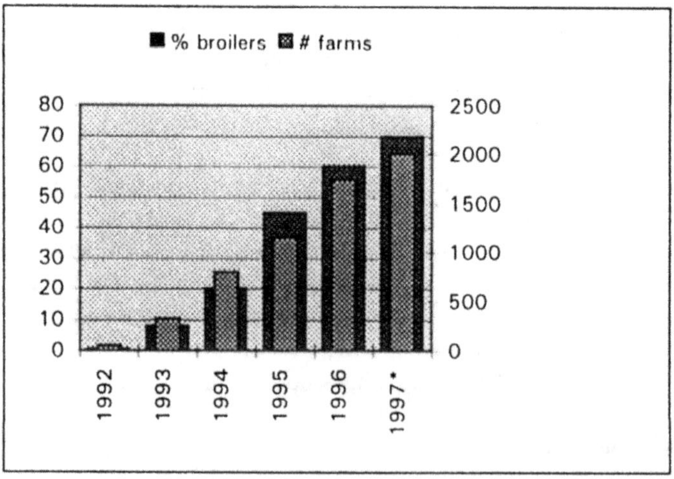

FIG. 3. IKB-PARTICIPATION BY NUMBER OF FARMS AND PERCENTAGE OF BROILER PRODUCTION CAPACITY

IKB Eggs

After a pilot period this scheme started in 1996. As with poultry the most important element was to give guarantees with regard to the microbiological quality of the product. There is participation in the scheme by about 15% of the total national egg production.

IKB Cattle

This redeveloped scheme started in the middle of 1996. The scheme covers the main elements of public concern: origin, traceability and (absence of) growth promotors. Against the background of the continuing consumer pressure within the EU with regard to maintaining the ban on growth promotors and the recent BSE-problem, it is expected that a large proportion of the cattle farmers and industry will participate. This scheme will also be used for the labelling of veal and beef, meeting the requirements of the EU-legislation. The labelling will be mandatory by January 2000.

COST/BENEFIT OF IKB

For the individual producer participation in IKB must be part of a long-term strategy. The most important benefit in the long run is a stronger competitive position in the market. As stated earlier, more and more customers are demanding products which are being produced in an QAS-production chain. That means that participating is in the end the only way to stay in business. Whether IKB will result in higher prices is difficult to predict; however, IKB does result in lower production costs for the producer (less veterinary drugs, better growth, better feed conversion and lower incidence of inspection abnormalities), but perhaps the most important profit is that participation in IKB makes a producer more competitive. It forces the producer constantly to improve himself and to anticipate new developments. And that innovative attitude is necessary to survive the fierce competition in this industry.

IKB IN AN INTERNATIONAL PERSPECTIVE

Development of IKB-systems are taking place in many other countries, e.g. Denmark, Germany, UK, France. It is very interesting, but difficult to make comparisons between these developments. Some systems only exist on paper.

An IKB-type system must prove itself in practice and not through nice brochures. In that respect, the most advanced IKB-systems are presently operating in industry, systems which have been tested in practice and among a great number of participants.

FUTURE DEVELOPMENTS

IKB means a market-oriented production. Therefore an IKB-scheme is a dynamic system. The industry has to continuously investigate whether changes in the basic IKB-scheme are necessary to serve the market even better. In this regard, aspects such as animal welfare, environment, hygiene and pathogens need to be mentioned. Furthermore, it can be seen that IKB is used by individual companies as a basis for further developments. A good example in this respect is opening the Japanese and Korean markets to Dutch pork. The IKB-approach proved to be very suitable to fulfil the very strict guarantees the Japanese and Korean markets demand for the quality of imported pork.

CONCLUSION

In the near future the meat industry will survive the intense international competition with only the optimum market-oriented approach to satisfy consumer demands. Therefore, a strict quality assurance approach for all parts of the production process, from conception to consumption, is absolutely necessary. With the development of the IKB-schemes the Dutch meat industry has made a first but important step towards this goal.

REFERENCES

CANDEL, M.J.J.M., SCHIFFERSTEIN, H.M.J. and van TRIJP, J.C.M. 1998. Comprehensive approach to image research: an illustration for fresh meat products in the Netherlands. Tijdschrift voor Sociaal-Wetenschappelijk Onderzoek voor de Land- en Tuinbouw. Submitted.

PVV 1997. Statistische jaarrapport 1996, rapportnr 9712a [Statistical annual report].

PVV 1997. Jaarverslag 1996. [Annual report 1996].

PPE 1997. Voortgang IKB-deelnemers, SV/26.06.97/3.5.

INDEX